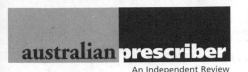

australian **prescriber**

An Independent Review

P9-DIZ-776

Pharmacokinetics
Made Easy

Donald J Birkett

The McGraw-Hill Companies, Inc.

Sydney New York San Francisco Auckland
Bangkok Bogotá Caracas Hong Kong
Kuala Lumpur Lisbon London Madrid
Mexico City Milan New Delhi San Juan
Seoul Singapore Taipei Toronto

McGraw·Hill Australia

A Division of The McGraw·Hill Companies

Reprinted 1999

National Library of Australia Cataloguing-in-Publication data:

Birkett, D J (Donald John).
Pharmacokinetics made easy.

ISBN 0 07 470 609 8.

1. Pharmacokinetics. I. Title.

615.7

Published in Australia by
McGraw-Hill Book Company Australia Pty Limited
4 Barcoo Street, Roseville NSW 2069, Australia
Acquisitions Editor: Kristen Baragwanath
Supervising Editor: Anna Crago
Editor: Tiffany Hutton, Indigo Ink
Cover design: Jacqui Spedding
Designed and typeset by Indigo Ink
Illustrator: Alan Laver
Printed in Hong Kong by Hilwing Printing Co.

FOREWORD

Australian Prescriber is the national therapeutics bulletin. It is an independently edited review of therapeutics. This independent status allows *Australian Prescriber* to review issues which may receive little attention in other publications.

One topic which receives little coverage is pharmacokinetics. Although it can be a complex subject, an understanding of pharmacokinetics is essential if drugs are to be prescribed appropriately.

The Executive Editorial Board of *Australian Prescriber* recognised the lack of easily understood information about pharmacokinetics and decided to commission a series of articles to explain some of the parameters. Professor Don Birkett was commissioned to produce articles which would be helpful to readers who were not pharmacologists. The result was the 'Pharmacokinetics Made Easy' series which was published over several years in *Australian Prescriber*.

The series has been popular with requests for copies of the articles coming from around the world. The articles have been used in teaching medicine and related disciplines and have also been helpful to doctors studying for higher professional qualifications, for example in anaesthetics.

In response to these requests, the Executive Editorial Board decided that the series should be published as a booklet. There has been tremendous interest in this project from teachers of pharmacology around Australia, so I hope *Pharmacokinetics Made Easy* will become a standard textbook.

Dr John S Dowden
Editor, *Australian Prescriber*
Canberra

CONTENTS

PREFACE

Gone are the days when all patients received the same dose of a drug regardless of size, shape, sex, race and the presence of disease states and drug interactions. Clinical pharmacokinetics provides the means to prescribe the right dose for each patient, and this book provides a simple guide to the basics of clinical pharmacokinetics. Traditionally, pharmacokinetics was based on the abstract mathematical modelling of the time course of drug concentrations. Over the last 10 to 15 years, however, a physiologically based approach has been taken, which allows the direct application of the concepts to clinical situations, and to the prediction of the effects of disease processes, drug interactions and other factors that affect drug treatment. It brings the subject alive, and applies it to real patients and real clinical situations.

Some time ago, the Executive Editorial Board of *Australian Prescriber* asked me if I would write a series of articles outlining in a simple fashion the basic principles of clinical pharmacokinetics. The articles were to be understandable to family practitioners, take an applied approach using clinical examples, contain as few equations as possible, and be succinct. Over a period of nearly 10 years, 12 articles were written covering the important aspects of pharmacokinetics. These were closely edited by the Executive Editorial Board who ruthlessly curbed my inclination to include too many equations and material that was not directly relevant or easily understandable.

Whenever I give lectures in Australia and overseas, I am surprised how many people ask when the next article will appear or for copies of those already published. The articles have clearly been found useful in the teaching of health professionals and students in a variety of contexts. My own experience as a teacher is that there is no other readily available text or single source of material that deals with the subject simply, comprehensively and at an appropriate and practical level. It seemed it would be useful, therefore, to make the articles accessible in one volume — this small book is the result.

The book describes the physiological processes that determine the fundamental pharmacokinetic parameters — clearance and volume of distribution. It shows how this information can be used to predict the effects of drug interactions and disease states on steady state drug concentrations and therefore effects. The factors determining the time course of drug concentrations and effects after single and multiple doses are described, and the concepts used to develop a rational approach to the design of dosage regimens and therapeutic drug monitoring. Illustrations, usually based on clinical examples, are included throughout to aid understanding. Equations are presented as a way of describing the basic physiological factors which determine the various pharmacokinetic parameters. This is emphasised in the early part of the book by writing most of the equations in words rather than symbols.

In revising the articles for publication in book form, I have added, both for completeness and to aid understanding, some material which was originally precluded because of space requirements in the journal. A glossary of the symbols used and a list of the important equations also have been added. At the end of each chapter, self-assessment questions have been included to test understanding of the principles involved.

My thanks go to the editor of *Australian Prescriber*, Dr John Dowden, and to the members of the Executive Editorial Board of the journal. The former pursued me relentlessly for the next article in the series, and both, by their sensible editing, kept the articles as close as possible to the original concept. The final product reflects their efforts as well as my own.

I also thank Karen Lillywhite who produced the references from which the figures were drawn, and Heather Aubert who typed the manuscript.

Don Birkett
25 April 1998

ABOUT THE AUTHORS

Don Birkett obtained his medical degree from Sydney University in 1967 and a D Phil in Biochemistry from Oxford University in 1970. He has been Professor and Head of Clinical Pharmacology at Flinders University of South Australia and Flinders Medical Centre since 1977. His major research interest has been in the field of drug metabolism using techniques ranging from *in vitro* molecular biological methods to *in vivo* pharmacokinetic studies. He was Chair of the International Union of Pharmacology (IUPHAR) Section on Drug Metabolism from 1994 to 1998. He has played a significant role in drug regulation, being a past member of the Australian Drug Evaluation Committee, and the current Chair of the Pharmaceutical Benefits Advisory Committee which considers the listing of drugs for government subsidy in Australia. He also currently chairs the Australian Drug Utilization Subcommittee and the WHO Working Group on Drug Statistics Methodology. He has published more than 220 scientific papers and books.

He has been teaching clinical pharmacology, pharmacology and pharmacokinetics for more than 25 years to medical and science students, and to drug regulators and members of the pharmaceutical industry.

Australian Prescriber is an independently edited review of therapeutics. The journal was launched by the Australian Department of Health in 1975. Since then it has gained an international reputation for its articles on drugs and drug treatments. The quality of the content is set by an editorial board of practising clinicians assisted by an advisory panel drawn from the leading Australasian medical colleges and societies.

Australian Prescriber has a circulation of almost 60,000 people. It is sent to doctors, dentists and pharmacists and provided to students of these disciplines through their training institutions. Most of the readers are in Australia, but there is a growing readership in the Asia–Pacific region. *Australian Prescriber* was a founder member of the International Society of Drug Bulletins. It was also one of the first medical journals to make its full text available online. (http://www.australianprescriber.com)

DEFINITIONS AND UNITS OF SYMBOLS

Symbol	Units	Definition
A	mg	amount of drug in body
AUC	mg*hour/L	total area under the plasma drug concentration-time curve
AUC_{iv}	mg*hour/L	area under the plasma drug concentration-time curve after an IV dose
AUC_{oral}	mg*hour/L	area under the plasma drug concentration-time curve after an oral dose
C	mg/L	concentration of drug in plasma
C_0	mg/L	concentration of drug in plasma after a single dose extrapolated back to zero time
C_b	mg/L	concentration of drug in blood
CL	L/hour	total clearance of drug from plasma
CL_{CR}	L/hour	creatinine clearance
CL_{GF}	L/hour	renal drug clearance by glomerular filtration
CL_H	L/hour	hepatic clearance of drug from plasma
CL_{int}	L/hour	intrinsic clearance of drug in an organ of elimination
CL_R	L/hour	renal clearance of drug
CL_S	L/hour	renal drug clearance by tubular secretion
C_{max}	mg/L	maximum plasma drug concentration during a dosing interval
C_{min}	mg/L	minimum plasma drug concentration during a dosing interval

Symbol	Units	Definition
C_{ss}	mg/L	concentration of drug in plasma at steady state during a constant-rate intravenous infusion
C_u	mg/L	unbound drug concentration in plasma
DR	mg/hour	dosing rate
E	ratio	extraction ratio for an organ
E_H	ratio	hepatic extraction ratio
EC_{50}	mg/L	concentration giving one-half the maximum effect
E_{max}	varies	maximum effect
F	ratio	bioavailability of drug
f_e	ratio	fraction of drug systemically available that is excreted unchanged in urine
f_g	ratio	fraction of an oral dose that is absorbed intact into the portal circulation
f_H	ratio	fraction of drug entering the liver that escapes extraction
fm	ratio	fraction of drug systemically available that is converted to a metabolite
FR	ratio	fraction of drug reaching the renal tubular fluid that is reabsorbed
fu	ratio	fraction of drug unbound in plasma
fu_T	ratio	fraction of drug unbound in tissues
GFR	L/hour	glomerular filtration rate
k	/hour	elimination rate constant
K_a	mM	association constant for the binding of drug to protein
K_m	mg/L	Michaelis-Menten constant
λ (lambda)	ratio	ratio of concentration of drug in whole blood to that in plasma
P_u	mM	concentration of protein that does not bind drug

Symbol	Units	Definition
Q_H	L/hour	hepatic blood flow (portal vein plus hepatic artery)
τ (tau)	hour	dosing interval
V	L	volume of distribution (apparent) based on drug concentration in plasma
v	mg/hour	velocity of enzyme reaction (conversion of drug to metabolite)
V_{max}	mg/hour	maximal rate of enzyme reaction at saturating substrate concentration
V_p	L	plasma volume
V_T	L	physiologic volume outside plasma into which drug distributes

EQUATIONS

$Elimination\ rate\ =\ CL*C$ Equation 1.2

$DR\ =\ CL*C_{ss}$ Equation 1.4

$CL\ =\ \dfrac{dose}{AUC}$ Equation 1.6

$C_b = C*\lambda$ Equation 1.7

$V\ =\ \dfrac{A}{C}$ Equation 2.1

$V\ =\ V_p + \dfrac{fu}{fu_T}*V_T$ Equation 2.2

$loading\ dose\ =\ V*C$ Equation 2.3

$C_t\ =\ C_0*e^{-kt}$ Equation 3.1

$t_{\frac{1}{2}} = \dfrac{0.693}{k}$ Equation 3.2

$t_{\frac{1}{2}} = \dfrac{0.693*V}{CL}$ Equation 3.3

$k = \dfrac{CL}{V}$ Equation 3.4

$CL_H = Q_H * E_H$ Equation 4.1

$E_H = \dfrac{fu*CL_{int}}{Q_H + fu*CL_{int}}$ Equation 4.3

$CL_{int} = \dfrac{V_{max}}{K_m}$ Equation 4.4

$$CL_H = Q_H * \frac{fu * CL_{int}}{Q_H + fu * CL_{int}}$$

Equation 4.5

$$F = f_g * f_H$$

Equation 5.1

$$(f_H = 1 - E_H \qquad \text{Equation 6.6})$$

$$F = \frac{AUC_{oral}}{AUC_{iv}}$$

Equation 5.5

$$CL = CL_R + CL_H$$

Equation 6.1

$$f_e = \frac{CL_R}{CL}$$

Equation 6.2

$$CL_R = fu \, (GFR + CL_s)(1 - FR)$$

Equation 7.3

$$CL_{CR} = \frac{(140 - age)(weight \ in \ kg)}{814 * serum \ creatinine \ (mmol \, / \, L)}$$

Equation from fn 1, p 63

$$fu = \frac{C_u}{C}$$

Equation 8.2

$$C_{ss} = \frac{F * DR}{CL}$$

Equation 9.1

$$\frac{C_{max} \, steady \ state}{C_{max} \, first \ dose} = \frac{1}{1 - e^{-k\tau}}$$

Equation 11.3

$$\frac{C_{max} \, steady \ state}{C_{min} \, steady \ state} = \frac{1}{e^{-k\tau}}$$

Equation 11.4

1

CLEARANCE

The two primary pharmacokinetic parameters are clearance (CL) and volume of distribution (V). They are primary parameters in that they are determined by, and can be described in terms of, fundamental physiological processes. The third important pharmacokinetic parameter, half-life, is a composite parameter derived from the clearance and volume of distribution.

What is clearance?

'Clearance' describes the efficiency of irreversible elimination of a drug from the body. Elimination in this context refers either to the excretion of the unchanged drug into urine, gut contents, expired air, sweat, etc, or to the metabolic conversion of the drug into a different chemical compound, predominantly in the liver, but also to some extent in other organs. When the drug has been metabolised, the parent drug has been cleared or eliminated, even though the metabolite may still be in the body. Uptake of the drug into tissues is not clearance if the unchanged drug eventually comes back out of the tissue, however slowly this occurs.

Clearance is defined as 'the volume of blood cleared of drug per unit time' and the units are thus volume per time, usually litres per hour or mL per minute. We can refer to clearance by a particular organ, such as liver or kidney, by a particular metabolic pathway, or by the whole body. Total body clearance is the sum of all the different clearance processes occurring for a given drug.

Let's consider an example. What does it mean if the clearance of a particular drug by the liver is 60 L/hour and liver blood flow is 90 L/hour? It does *not* mean that 60 L of blood going through the liver is totally cleared of the drug and the next 30 L is not cleared at all. Rather, it does mean that two-thirds (60/90) of the drug entering the liver in the blood is irreversibly removed by the liver (cleared) in one pass. The value of two-thirds for this drug is called the *extraction ratio* and is simply one minus the ratio of concentration of drug in blood *leaving* the liver to that in blood *entering* the liver.

$$extraction\ ratio = 1 - \frac{concentration\ out}{concentration\ in}$$

Equation 1.1

Obviously, the most drug that could be removed by the liver is all that enters the organ. In this case, the 'concentration out' would be 0.0, extraction ratio would be 1.0 and the hepatic clearance 90 L/hour. The further significance of the extraction ratio will be discussed in Chapter 4. For the present, it should be noted that the minimum clearance by an organ is zero and the maximum clearance by an organ is the blood flow to the organ.

Clearance and elimination rate

Another definition of clearance is that it is the constant relating the concentration of drug in the plasma to the elimination rate.

$$elimination\ rate = clearance\ (CL)*plasma\ drug\ concentration\ (C)$$
$$\ \ \ (mg/hour)\ \ \ \ \ \ \ \ \ \ (L/hour)\ \ \ \ \ \ \ \ \ \ \ \ \ \ \ \ \ \ \ (mg/L)$$

Equation 1.2

It is apparent that for a given clearance, which is a constant characteristic of a particular drug and a particular patient, the elimination rate varies directly with the plasma drug concentration.

Why is clearance important?

Clearance is the one parameter that determines the maintenance dose rate required to achieve a target plasma concentration (and therefore effect) at steady state. Steady state is defined as the situation at which the rate of drug administration is equal to the rate of drug elimination so that the amount of drug in the body, and therefore the plasma drug concentration, remains constant. At steady state,

---

elimination rate = maintenance dose rate (DR)

Equation 1.3

From Equations 1.2 and 1.3, the maintenance dose rate required to achieve a target steady state plasma drug concentration can be calculated as:

---

maintenance dose rate (DR) = clearance (CL)*steady state drug
concentration (C_{ss})

(mg/hour)   *(L/hour)*   *(mg/L)*

Equation 1.4

This is illustrated in Figure 1.1 (following page) for constant rate intravenous infusions of two drugs, for one of which the clearance is double that of the other. Note that, with a constant infusion, the plasma drug concentration rises steadily until it eventually reaches a plateau or steady state when the rate of drug administration equals the rate of drug elimination.

The oral dosing situation is slightly more complex because the drug concentration fluctuates during the dosing interval as the drug is absorbed and eliminated. Eventually, however, the amount of drug eliminated during the dosing interval equals the dose administered, and the drug concentrations then fluctuate over the same range during each dosing interval; that is, steady state has been reached. At this point, the *average drug concentration over the dosing interval* is the same as the steady state plasma concentration for a constant intravenous infusion at the same dose rate. From Equation 1.4, it is easy to see that, *for a given dose rate, the plasma drug concentration is inversely proportional to clearance.* For example, if the clearance is reduced by half, the steady state concentration will double (see Figure 1.1).

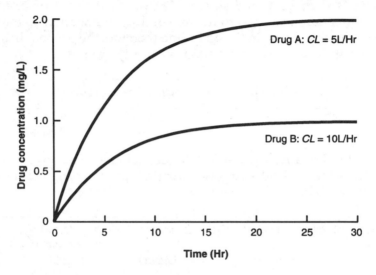

Figure 1.1: Effect of clearance on steady state drug concentration

Clearance determines the plasma drug concentration at steady state. For both drugs A and B, the dose rate is 10 mg/hour.

How is clearance measured?

The classical method of measuring *renal* clearance (for example, of creatinine or drugs) is to measure the rate of excretion in urine, and the blood concentration at the same time. This is the well-known $CL = U*V/P$ relationship where U is urine drug concentration, V is urine flow rate and P is the plasma (or blood) concentration of a solute such as creatinine or a drug. This is actually the same as Equation 1.2, as $U*V$ is the excretion rate of the solute.

To obtain *total body* clearance of a drug, we can use Equation 1.4 to obtain clearance from the steady state drug concentration during a constant intravenous infusion.

$$clearance = \frac{dose\ rate}{steady\ state\ plasma\ concentration}$$

$$CL = \frac{DR}{C_{ss}}$$

Equation 1.5

Alternatively, we can take frequent blood samples after a single intravenous dose, measure the drug concentration in each, and calculate the area under the drug concentration versus time curve (AUC) (see Figure 1.2 on following page). Then:

$$clearance = \frac{dose}{AUC}$$

$$(L\ /\ hour) \qquad \frac{mg}{mg*hour\ /\ L}$$

Equation 1.6

From this relationship, it can be seen that the total area under the plasma concentration time curve after a single dose is, like the steady state concentration, only determined by the dose and the clearance.

Plasma or blood drug concentrations?

It is the convention in pharmacokinetics to use *plasma* concentrations of drugs as this is what is usually measured in the laboratory. Measuring whole blood concentrations tends to be more difficult due to the presence of more interfering compounds. Therefore, throughout this book, pharmacokinetic parameters will be referred to in terms of plasma drug concentrations. It should be remembered, however, that the tissues and eliminating organs such as the kidneys and liver are perfused with blood, not plasma. The plasma concentration of a drug can be related to the whole blood concentration by the blood:plasma concentration ratio (λ).

$$\lambda = \frac{drug\ concentration\ in\ whole\ blood}{drug\ concentration\ in\ plasma} = \frac{C_b}{C}$$

$$C_b = C * \lambda$$

Equation 1.7

This ratio is usually close to 1.0 as the drug concentrations in the cellular and plasma components of blood are usually about the same. The ratio cannot be less than about 0.5 (the haematocrit). It can, however, be quite large for highly lipophilic

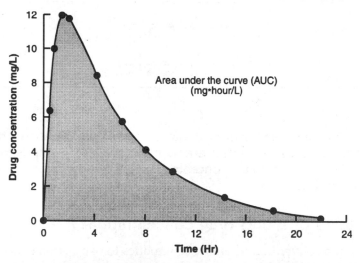

Figure 1.2: Measurement of clearance

Clearance can be determined by measuring plasma drug concentrations at multiple times after a single intravenous dose.

$$CL(L/hour) = \frac{Dose\ (mg)}{AUC(mg * hour/L)}$$

drugs like cyclosporin and chloroquine which are relatively concentrated in the red cells. In such cases, it is better to express clearance and volume of distribution in terms of drug concentrations in whole blood rather than in plasma.

Summary

Clearance is the primary pharmacokinetic parameter that is a measure of the efficiency of drug elimination and therefore, for any given dose, determines the plasma drug concentration and effect at steady state during constant dosing.

Self-test questions

1. Elimination of a drug refers to:
   a) excretion of its breakdown products in the urine
   b) renal excretion of the unchanged drug
   c) uptake of drug from the blood into the liver
   d) metabolism of the drug in the liver
   e) distribution of the drug into fat

2. The elimination rate of a drug is:
   a) a constant for a particular drug and patient
   b) the extent to which it is excreted in urine
   c) directly proportional to the plasma drug concentration
   d) directly proportional to the clearance
   e) the extent to which the drug is excreted in the faeces

3. Clearance:
   a) depends on the elimination rate
   b) refers to the efficiency of elimination of drug by an organ or the whole body
   c) cannot be greater than blood flow to an organ
   d) determines the steady state drug concentration during constant dosing
   e) is determined by the half-life

4. Two definitions of clearance are:

   a) the volume of blood or plasma irreversibly cleared of drug per unit time

   b) the time taken to reduce the plasma concentration by half

   c) the constant relating the rate of elimination of a drug to the plasma drug concentration

   d) the amount of drug metabolised per unit time

   e) the amount of drug excreted in urine per unit time

2

VOLUME OF DISTRIBUTION

Volume of distribution is one of the two major independent pharmacokinetic parameters. The other (clearance) was dealt with in Chapter 1.

What is volume of distribution (V)?

It is not a real 'volume'. It is the parameter relating the concentration of a drug in the plasma to the total amount of the drug in the body. For example, if a drug has a plasma concentration of 10 mg/L when there is 1000 mg of the drug in the body, the volume of distribution would be 100 L, that is, dissolving 1000 mg of drug in an imaginary volume of 100 L would give a concentration of 10 mg/L.

$$V = \frac{total\ amount\ of\ drug\ in\ body\ (A)}{plasma\ drug\ concentration\ (C)}$$

Equation 2.1

If volume of distribution is an 'imaginary' volume, what is it determined by? The major determinant is the relative strength of binding of the drug to tissue components as compared with plasma proteins. If a drug is very tightly bound by tissues and not by blood, most of the drug in the body will be held in the tissues and very little in the plasma, so that the drug will appear to be dissolved in a large volume and V will be large. Examples of such drugs are the lipid soluble bases such as imipramine and chlorpromazine. Conversely, if the drug is tightly bound to plasma proteins and not to tissues, V can be very close to blood volume as is the case for warfarin. This can be summarised by the following expression which shows that the main determinant of V is the ratio of binding in plasma to the binding in tissues (fu/fu_T).

$$V = plasma\ Volume\ (V) + \frac{fraction\ unbound\ in\ plasma\ (fu)}{fraction\ unbound\ in\ tissue\ (fu_T)} * Tissue\ volume\ (V_T)$$

Equation 2.2

Some examples of volumes of distribution are:

- warfarin 8 L
- digoxin 420 L
- theophylline 35 L
- imipramine 2100 L
- quinidine 150 L

How is V measured?

The simplest method is illustrated in Figure 2.1.

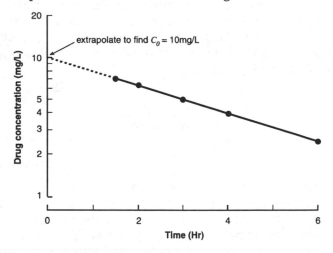

Figure 2.1: Determination of volume of distribution

A dose of 200 mg was given and the first sample taken 1½ hours later. Note that the drug concentration scale is logarithmic (see Chapter 3).

$$V = \frac{Amount\ of\ drug\ in\ body}{Plasma\ drug\ concentration}$$

At zero time:

$$V = \frac{dose}{C_0} = \frac{200}{10} = 20L$$

In this case, a dose of 200 mg of a drug is given at time zero, blood samples collected and the plasma drug concentrations measured. When the logarithm of drug concentration is plotted against time, a straight line results. If this is extrapolated back to zero time, it gives the plasma drug concentration before any drug is eliminated, that is, when the whole dose (200 mg) is still in the body. In this case, the extrapolated concentration at zero time is 10 mg/L and V is 20 L (200 mg/ 10 mg/L).

What is V used for?

In the previous chapter, we saw that clearance determines the drug concentration at steady state during continuous administration. If we just start with the maintenance dose, it takes some time to accumulate to steady state. To get close to steady state more quickly, a *loading dose* is often used and V is the determinant of the size of the loading dose. In the example given above, if we want to get quickly to 10 mg/L, we have to give enough drug to give a concentration of 10 mg/L when 'dissolved' in the 20 L volume of distribution — a loading dose of 200 mg in this example. The loading dose is given to 'fill up' the volume of distribution. Thus:

> *loading dose = V*target plasma concentration*
>
> *200 mg = 20 L*10 mg/L*

Equation 2.3

An example is calculating the loading dose of theophylline at the start of a theophylline infusion. The V of theophylline averages 0.5 L/kg (35 L in a 70 kg patient) so that the loading dose to achieve a plasma concentration of 10 mg/L (at the lower end of the therapeutic range) is 0.5 L/kg * 10 mg/L = 5 mg/kg or 350 mg in this patient. As the actual range of V in a number of patients is 0.3–0.7 L/kg, the actual concentration could be in the range 7–17 mg/L. The effect of a loading dose is illustrated in Figure 2.2.

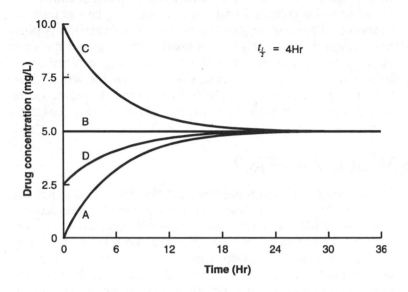

Figure 2.2: Use of a loading dose

With no loading dose, drug accumulates slowly to steady state (dose A). Loading dose B happened to give an initial concentration the same as that maintained by the infusion which followed the loading dose. Loading dose C was overestimated and D underestimated. The initial concentrations in C and D are closer to the steady state concentration, but it still takes the same time to reach steady state.

Is the rate of distribution from blood to tissues important?

A drug is either injected directly into the blood, or absorbed from the gut or other administration site into the blood, so that the immediate volume of distribution is blood volume and concentrations are initially high. The drug then distributes from the blood into various tissues at a rate and to an extent which depends on the perfusion of the tissue and the ease with which the drug can pass through the lipid membranes of the cells.

Some tissues such as the brain are highly perfused and drugs such as diazepam and thiopentone distribute very rapidly from the blood into them. Distribution to less highly perfused tissues such as skeletal muscle and fat occurs more slowly.

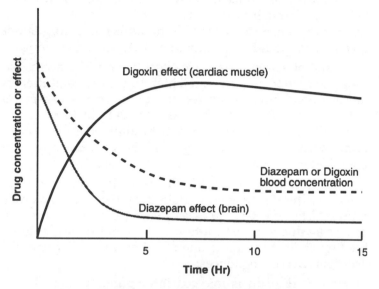

Figure 2.3: Drugs with slow distribution phases

Plasma drug concentration falls rapidly initially due to redistribution and then more slowly due to elimination. The effect of diazepam is in a highly perfused tissue (brain). The site of action of digoxin is a compartment to which the drug is distributed slowly. Once the distribution phase is over, effects of both drugs are related to plasma concentration.

Figure 2.3 illustrates how this can have opposite effects depending on whether the site of action of a drug is in a rapidly or slowly perfused tissue. Diazepam and digoxin have rather similar distribution characteristics, with blood concentrations falling relatively rapidly over 4–6 hours as the drug is redistributed from the blood and highly perfused tissues into tissues such as muscle and fat. Both then have slow elimination phases with half-lives of 1–2 days.

Consider the following examples:

1. *Diazepam used intravenously in status epilepticus.* The site of action is the brain which is highly perfused so that brain diazepam concentrations *and anticonvulsant effect* follow blood diazepam concentrations. Concentrations *and effect* fall rapidly initially due to redistribution to other tissues and fitting can recur within 2–4 hours if more drug is not given, even though the elimination half-life is very long.

   If the site of action for a toxic effect is a rapidly accessible tissue compartment, the initial high concentrations after an intravenous bolus before redistribution occurs can cause serious toxic effects. In this case, the rate of intravenous injection must be slowed down to allow distribution to occur while the drug is being administered. Examples are the intravenous use of theophylline and lignocaine.

2. *Digoxin given intravenously.* In this case, digoxin distributes slowly to the site of action (inotropic effect) in the cardiac muscle. The effect *increases* as plasma concentrations are *decreasing* due to redistribution of digoxin into less accessible tissues, including the site of action in cardiac muscle. This has two consequences:

   a) Even if digoxin is injected intravenously, it will take about 6 hours to exert the full effect, giving no advantage of intravenous over oral administration. Therefore, loading with digoxin is best carried out with divided oral doses at least 6 hours apart so that the full effect of each dose can be assessed before more is given.

   b) In the first 6–8 hours after administration, digoxin plasma concentrations bear no relationship to effect. Samples for plasma concentration monitoring must therefore always be taken at least 6 hours after a dose and preferably at the end of the dosing interval just before the next dose.

Summary

The volume of distribution is the constant relating the amount of drug in the body to the plasma drug concentration. Its major physiological determinant is the ratio between the strength of binding of the drug to plasma proteins and the strength of binding to tissue components. It is the pharmacokinetic parameter used to calculate the loading dose of a drug. The rate of distribution from or to the site of action can be the determinant of the onset or offset of drug effects.

Self-test questions

1. Volume of distribution is:
   a) the total volume of the body
   b) the volume of extracellular fluid
   c) equal to the volume of total body water
   d) the constant relating amount of drug in the body to the plasma drug concentration
   e) the volume of the body minus the blood volume

2. The loading dose of a drug is determined by:
   a) the clearance
   b) the elimination rate
   c) the target plasma drug concentration
   d) the volume of distribution
   e) the molecular weight of the drug

3. The rate of distribution of a drug can determine:
   a) the volume of distribution
   b) the onset of drug effect
   c) the rate of drug elimination
   d) the duration of drug effect
   e) the clearance

4. Volume of distribution can be measured using:
   a) the plasma drug concentration extrapolated back to zero time after administration
   b) the rate of elimination at a particular time after the dose
   c) the clearance
   d) the rate of onset of drug effect
   e) the duration of drug effect

3

HALF-LIFE

What is half-life?

Half-life is the time taken for the amount of drug in the body (or the plasma concentration) to fall by half. The elimination of a drug is usually an exponential (logarithmic) process so that a constant proportion of the drug in the body is eliminated per unit time. This is illustrated in Figure 3.1 on the following page on both linear and semi-logarithmic graphs. When plotted as a logarithm of plasma concentration versus time, a straight line results. This is known as 'first order elimination'.

Elimination rate constant

The fall in plasma drug concentration after a single dose is an exponential (logarithmic) function of the time after dose, and is described by the expression:

$$C_t = C_0 * e^{-kt}$$

Equation 3.1

In this expression C_t is the concentration at various times (t) after the dose, C_0 is the initial concentration at time zero and k is the elimination rate constant. In Chapter 1, we saw that the elimination rate is the *amount* of drug eliminated per unit time and has the units 'mg/hour'. The elimination rate constant is a proportionality constant expressing the *proportion* of drug in the body eliminated per unit time. It has the units 'per hour'. For example, when the elimination rate constant is 0.223, one-fifth of the drug in the body is eliminated per hour.

How does the elimination rate constant relate to the half-life?

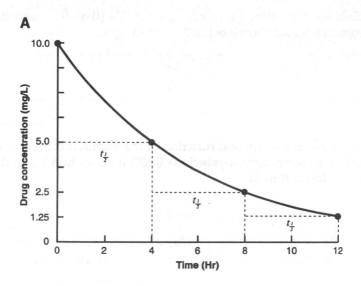

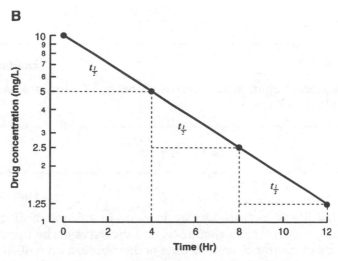

Figure 3.1: Time course of drug elimination

First order elimination of a drug with a half-life of 4 hours plotted on (A) a linear scale and (B) a semi-logarithmic scale. The plasma concentration falls by half each half-life.

Solving Equation 3.1 when $C_t = 0.5*C_0$ (that is, when the plasma concentration has fallen by half) gives:

$$k = \frac{0.693}{t_{1/2}}$$

Equation 3.2

Half-life is a reciprocal function of the elimination rate constant. The seemingly mysterious 0.693 in Equation 3.2 is the natural logarithm of 2.

What determines half-life?

Half-life is a composite pharmacokinetic parameter determined by both clearance (CL) and volume of distribution (V).

$$t_{1/2} = \frac{0.693*V}{CL}$$

Equation 3.3

and from Equation 3.2, the relationship of elimination rate constant to V and CL is:

$$k = \frac{CL}{V}$$

Equation 3.4

Half-life is increased by an increase in volume of distribution or a decrease in clearance, and vice versa. The opposing effects of clearance and volume of distribution on half-life are illustrated in Table 3.1 by reference to a number of commonly used drugs. For example, ethosuximide and flucytosine have the same volume of distribution, but their half-lives are 10-fold different due to a 10-fold difference in clearance. By contrast, digoxin and flucytosine have the same clearance, but the half-lives are different because of the 10-fold difference in volume of distribution. Chloroquine has a high clearance, but a very long half-life because of the very large volume of distribution due to the high lipid solubility of the drug and the resulting extensive binding in adipose and other tissues.

Table 3.1: Effects of clearance and volume of distribution in determining half-life

Drug	Clearance (L/hour)	Volume of distribution (L)	Half-life (hours)
Ethosuximide	0.7	49	48.0
Flucytosine	8.0	49	4.2
Digoxin	7.0	420	40.0
Morphine	63.0	280	3.0
Haloperidol	46.0	1,400	20.0
Chloroquine	45.0	12,950	200.0

It is easy enough to understand why a change in clearance would change half-life. A decrease in the efficiency of elimination would be expected to increase the time taken to eliminate the drug. But why should the volume of distribution also determine half-life? The larger the volume of distribution, the more the drug is concentrated in the tissues compared to the blood. It is drug in the blood that is exposed to hepatic or renal clearance, so that when the distribution volume is large, these mechanisms have less drug to work on. By contrast, if the volume of distribution is small, most of the drug in the body is in the blood and is accessible to the elimination processes.

In disease states such as renal or hepatic failure, clearance and volume of distribution can sometimes change in the same direction, exerting opposing effects on half-life which may, therefore, not change, although clearance is decreased. Half-life is therefore not a good measure of changes in the efficiency of elimination (clearance) of drugs.

Why is half-life important?

Half-life is a major determinant of:

- *The duration of action after a single dose*. After a single dose, the longer the half-life the longer the plasma concentration will stay in the effective range. However, the duration of action is a logarithmic, not linear, function of the dose so that increasing the dose is an inefficient way of increasing the duration of action. A simple rule of thumb is that doubling the dose increases the duration of action by one half-life.

- *The time required to reach steady state with chronic dosing*. With a constant rate infusion, the accumulation of drug to steady state is a mirror image of the elimination when dosing is stopped. The approach to steady state in terms of half-lives is shown in Table 3.2.

Table 3.2: Accumulation to steady state

Number of half-lives since starting constant rate dosing	Plasma concentration as a percentage of eventual steady state concentration (%)
1	50
2	75
3	87.5
4	93.75
5	96.875

It can be seen that it takes 3–5 half-lives to reach the target plasma concentration (approximate steady state). From Table 3.1, it can be seen that it will take about 16 hours to reach steady state with flucytosine, 12 hours with morphine, 160 hours (7 days) with digoxin, and about 5 weeks with chloroquine. This is why chloroquine prophylaxis must be started some weeks before the patient goes to a malarious area.

The importance of these considerations can also be seen in relation to monitoring theophylline plasma concentrations during an aminophylline infusion. The theophylline half-life may be as long as 20 hours in patients with severe cardiac failure and/or liver disease. A plasma concentration measured 20 hours after starting an infusion will only be 50% of the concentration that will eventually be reached if the infusion is continued at the same rate, and this must be taken into account when considering adjustments to the infusion rate. Even when a loading dose is given before the infusion, it still takes the same time to reach steady state, although the starting concentration is, of course, closer to the eventual steady state concentration (see Figure 2.2).

• *The dosing frequency required to avoid too large fluctuations in plasma concentration during the dosing interval.* With steady state dosing, the extent to which the plasma concentration fluctuates over the dosage interval is determined by the half-life and the time between doses. If a drug is given every half-life and is rapidly absorbed to reach a maximum (peak) concentration, then over one half-life the concentration will fall to half the peak concentration. That is, the peak concentrations will be double the trough (predose) concentrations and the fluctuation in plasma concentration over the dosage interval will be twofold. If a drug is given more

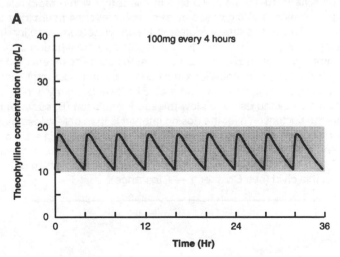

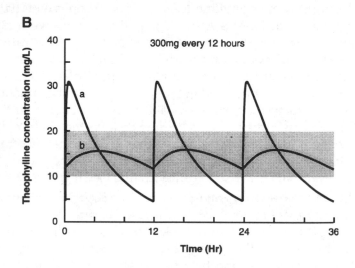

Figure 3.2: Fluctuation in plasma concentration during intermittent dosing

Effect of half-life and frequency of dosing on the fluctuation in plasma concentration over the dosing interval. The example shown is for theophylline treatment of a 20 kg child, who has a theophylline half-life of 4 hours, at a total daily dose of 600 mg. The therapeutic 'window' for theophylline is 10–20 mg/L. To stay in this range with a rapid release oral preparation, 100 mg doses must be given every 4 hours, day and night (A). This is because the plasma theophylline concentration falls by almost half (from 18.2 mg/L to 10.3 mg/L) over the 4 hour half-life. If the same preparation is given 12-hourly at the same dose rate (300 mg every 12 hours), concentrations fluctuate between 30.5 mg/L (toxic) and 4.4 mg/L (ineffective) (B, curve a). Effective 12-hourly dosing can be achieved by the use of a slow release formulation (B, curve b) because the fluctuation over the dosing interval is then determined by the absorption rate rather than the elimination rate. Note that in each case the AVERAGE concentration over the dosing interval is the same (14.7 mg/L) as this is determined only by the clearance which is 1.7 L/hour in this child (see Chapter 1 — Clearance).

frequently than every half-life, the fluctuations will be small. If the half-life is short and the drug shows dose-related toxicity, it is often difficult to dose frequently enough to avoid toxicity at the peaks, and lack of effect as the plasma concentration falls to low levels before the next dose. An example is theophylline therapy in children, who have theophylline half-lives as short as 2–5 hours. The therapeutic plasma concentration range for theophylline concentration is 10–20 mg/L, so a rapidly absorbed preparation would have to be given every 4 hours to stay within this range (Figure 3.2). As this is clearly impracticable, sustained-release formulations are used which ideally mimic a constant rate infusion. The fluctuation in plasma concentration is then determined by the slow *absorption* rate rather than the rapid *elimination* rate, and they can be given every 12 hours which is a much more feasible proposition.

Summary

Elimination rate constant is a proportionality constant expressing the proportion of drug in the body eliminated per unit time. Half-life is a reciprocal function of elimination rate constant and is determined by both clearance and volume of distribution. It determines the duration of action after a single dose of a drug, the time taken to reach steady state with constant dosing and the frequency with which doses can be given.

? Self-test questions

1. Half-life:
    a) is the time taken for the plasma concentration to fall by half
    b) has units of 'per hour'
    c) is the time taken for the amount of drug in the body to fall by half
    d) decreases as elimination rate constant increases
    e) increases as the elimination rate constant increases

2. Half-life:
   a) increases as clearance increases
   b) decreases as volume of distribution increases
   c) decreases as clearance increases
   d) increases as volume of distribution increases
   e) increases as elimination rate constant decreases

3. After a single dose of a drug which has a half-life of 12 hours, what percentage of the dose is still in the body after 1 day?
   a) 87.5%
   b) 75%
   c) 50%
   d) 25%
   e) 12.5%

4. During a constant rate intravenous infusion of a drug with an elimination rate constant of 0.173 per hour, the plasma drug concentration will be what percentage of steady state after 16 hours?
   a) 25%
   b) 50%
   c) 75%
   d) 87.5%
   e) 93.75%

5. Half-life determines:
   a) the loading dose
   b) the time to reach steady state
   c) the drug concentration at steady state during constant dosing
   d) the duration of action after a single dose
   e) the fluctuation in plasma drug concentration during a dosing interval

4

HOW DRUGS ARE CLEARED BY THE LIVER

The two major routes of drug elimination from the body are excretion as unchanged drug by the kidneys and elimination by metabolism in the liver. The balance between these depends on the relative efficiency of the two processes. For the current purpose, we will assume that the only method of clearance is by liver metabolism (this is essentially the case for many drugs) and consider the physiological factors which determine this process; that is, we are considering only hepatic clearance. In Chapter 7 the factors determining renal drug clearance will be looked at.

How hepatic extraction ratio and systemic clearance are related

In Chapter 1 we introduced the term 'hepatic extraction ratio', which is the fraction of the drug entering the liver in the blood which is irreversibly removed (extracted) during one pass of the blood through the liver. It is apparent that the extraction ratio could range from 0 (no drug at all is extracted) to 1.0 (all the drug entering the liver is extracted in one pass). This is illustrated in Figure 4.1.

It is intuitively obvious that clearance of drug by the liver will depend on the rate of delivery of drug to the liver (the hepatic blood flow) and on the efficiency of removal of drug which is presented to it (the extraction ratio). For example, consider the case of propranolol where 80% of the drug in the blood entering the liver is extracted in each pass (the extraction ratio is 0.8) and liver blood flow is 90 L/hour. Then 0.8 of 90 L of blood is cleared of propranolol each hour, that is, the hepatic clearance is 72 L/hour.

Put more generally,

$$hepatic\ clearance\ (CL_H) = hepatic\ blood\ flow\ (Q_H) * hepatic\ extraction\ ratio\ (E_H)$$

Equation 4.1

Thus, the two overall determinants of hepatic clearance are the efficiency of drug delivery in the blood (blood flow) and the efficiency of drug removal from the blood (extraction ratio). We now need to dissect further the extraction ratio term to see what determines how effectively the liver removes drug which is presented to it.

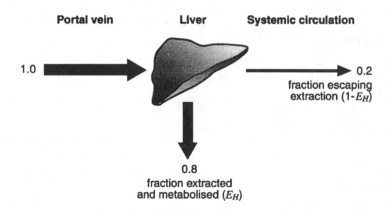

Figure 4.1: Hepatic extraction ratio

Bloody carrying drug enters the liver from the systemic circulation in the portal vein. In this example, the fraction extracted during each pass through the liver (E_H) is 0.8, so that 0.2 of the drug ($1-E_H$) survives to re-enter the systemic circulation from the hepatic vein. For a usual liver blood flow of 90 L/hour, the clearance of this drug would be 0.8*90 = 72L/hour

What determines hepatic extraction ratio

The equation describing the physiological parameters determining hepatic extraction ratio is as follows:

$$\text{extraction ratio} = \frac{\text{unbound fraction} * \text{intrinsic clearance}}{\text{blood flow} + \text{unbound fraction} * \text{intrinsic clearance}}$$

Equation 4.2

Expressed in symbols:

$$E_H = \frac{fu * CL_{int}}{Q_H + fu * CL_{int}}$$

Equation 4.3

Now let us consider what each of these terms means — we already know what hepatic blood flow (Q_H) is.

- *Unbound fraction (fu).* In some, but not all, circumstances the ability of the liver to remove drug depends on how tightly the drug is bound to proteins and cells in the blood. In general, it is only free (unbound) drug which is available for diffusion from the blood into the liver cell where metabolism takes place. The exceptions, drugs which are very highly extracted by the liver, will be discussed below. Protein binding of drugs is described further in Chapter 8.

- *Intrinsic clearance (CL_{int}).* This is the intrinsic ability of the liver to remove (metabolise) drug in the *absence* of restrictions imposed on drug delivery to the liver cell by blood flow and protein binding. It is what hepatic clearance would be if hepatic blood flow were unlimited and all the drug were unbound, and can have values many times higher than hepatic blood flow. In biochemical terms, it is really a measure of how active the liver drug metabolising enzymes are with that particular drug as substrate. Although intrinsic clearance can be very high, in fact many times greater than hepatic blood flow, it should be remembered that drug cannot be cleared more rapidly than it is presented to the liver, so that actual hepatic clearance cannot be higher than hepatic blood flow.

In molecular terms, intrinsic clearance is described by the parameters expressing the activity of a drug metabolising enzyme with a particular drug substrate.

$$CL_{int} = \frac{V_{max}}{K_m}$$

Equation 4.4

V_{max} is the maximal velocity of the reaction at saturating substrate concentration — the maximal rate at which the enzyme can convert the drug to a metabolite. K_m is the Michaelis constant and expresses how tightly the enzyme binds the drug substrate — the lower the K_m, the tighter the binding (it is a dissociation constant). We will return to Equation 4.4 when we consider non-linear pharmacokinetics in Chapter 9.

Simplifying the situation

From Equations 4.1 and 4.2 above, the full expression describing hepatic drug clearance is:

$$CL_H = Q_H * \frac{fu * CL_{int}}{Q_H + fu * CL_{int}}$$

Equation 4.5

This is complicated, and it is difficult to visualise what a change in one of the parameters would do to hepatic clearance. We can simplify matters by considering two limiting cases; one where the liver enzymes have very low activity towards a drug, and a second where the enzymes have very high activity.

The very low enzyme activity case

When the intrinsic clearance (enzyme activity) is much, much less than liver blood flow, Equation 4.5 cancels out as follows:

$$CL_H = \cancel{Q_H} * \frac{fu * CL_{int}}{\cancel{Q_H + fu*CL_{int}}}$$

Equation 4.6

This is because when $Q_H \gg fu*CL_{int}$, then $Q_H + fu*CL_{int}$ is approximately the same as Q_H. Then:

$$hepatic\ clearance = unbound\ fraction * intrinsic\ clearance$$

Equation 4.7

This is now a simple situation where we can say that clearance of such a drug by the liver is directly proportional to the degree of protein binding in the blood and the activity of the drug metabolising enzymes towards that particular drug. It does *not* depend on liver blood flow. As the capacity of the liver to remove drug is very limited, the liver is taking out drug as quickly as it can, even at low rates of delivery (blood flow). Increasing or decreasing the rate of supply by increasing or decreasing liver blood flow therefore makes little difference to the actual clearance. Such drugs are called capacity-limited, low hepatic clearance or low hepatic extraction ratio drugs. Diazepam is a good example.

The very high enzyme activity case

When the intrinsic clearance is much, much higher than liver blood flow, Equation 4.5 cancels out as follows:

$$CL_H = Q_H * \frac{\cancel{fu * CL_{int}}}{\cancel{Q_H} + fu*CL_{int}}$$

Equation 4.8

This is because when $fu*CL_{int} >> Q_H$, then $Q_H + fu*CL_{int}$ is approximately the same as $fu*CL_{int}$. Then:

> hepatic clearance = liver blood flow

Equation 4.9

The enzymes are so active that the liver removes all or nearly all the drug presented to it, so that the only thing determining the actual hepatic clearance is the rate of supply of drug to the liver (hepatic blood flow). As nearly all the drug is already being removed, changing the activity of the enzymes will make little or no difference. Even protein-bound drug can be stripped off in one pass, so that protein binding also is not important. These drugs are called flow-limited, high hepatic clearance or high hepatic extraction ratio drugs. Glyceryl trinitrate and verapamil are good examples.

Practical application of these concepts

We are now in a position to put these concepts to use in relation to specific drugs which are cleared mainly by metabolism. Simply by classifying a drug as having low or high hepatic extraction ratio and therefore clearance, we can know what physiological factors determine its hepatic clearance and thus its plasma concentrations and effects during maintenance dosing. Figure 4.2 shows the hepatic extraction ratio for a number of important drugs and summarises the physiological factors important in their hepatic clearance. For those who like looking at numbers, Table 4.1 shows how changes in intrinsic clearance or hepatic blood flow change the hepatic clearance of low and high hepatic extraction ratio drugs.

Systemic clearance and pre-systemic or first-pass extraction

So far, we have been dealing with systemic clearance, that is, clearance of drugs from the systemic circulation. Orally administered drugs are absorbed from the gut lumen into the portal circulation and must pass through the liver before reaching the systemic circulation. Pre-systemic or first-pass extraction refers to removal of drugs during this first pass through the liver during drug absorption. While the basic concepts are similar to those discussed in this chapter, there are important differences in the factors determining first-pass extraction of high extraction ratio drugs. Drug absorption, bioavailability and first-pass clearance are discussed in the next chapter.

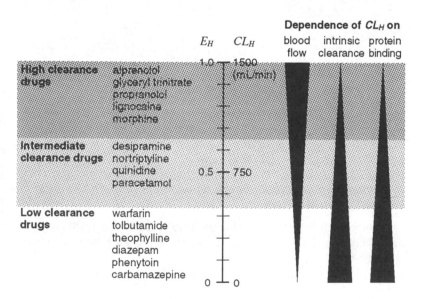

Figure 4.2: Determinants of hepatic extraction ratio and clearance

Hepatic extraction ratio and hepatic clearance of some important drugs. The major determinants of hepatic clearance and steady state plasma concentrations during maintenance dosing are illustrated.

Table 4.1: Effects of changes in hepatic blood flow and intrinsic clearance

| | Hepatic Extraction Ratio | | | |
| | Low | | High | |
	Initial	Changed	Initial	Changed
Halving $fu*CL_{int}$				
$fu*CL_{int}$ (L/hour)	5	2.5	1800	900
E_H	0.053	0.027	0.95	0.91
CL_H (L/hour)	4.7	2.4	86	82
Change in CL_H	49%		5%	
Halving Q_H				
Q_H (L/hour)	90	45	90	45
E_H	0.053	0.1	0.95	0.98
CL_H (L/hour)	4.7	4.5	86	44
Change in CL_H	4%		49%	

Hepatic blood flow is initially 90 L/hour and $fu*CL_{int}$ for the low and high extraction ratio drugs is initially 5 L/hour and 1800 L/hour respectively. The values shown were calculated using Equations 4.2 and 4.5. Possible changes in hepatic blood flow are physiologically relatively restricted (not more than about twofold) compared to the changes which can occur in CL_{int} or fu (10-fold or more).

Note the contrasting effects of changes in $fu*CL_{int}$ and Q_H on the hepatic extraction ratios and hepatic clearances of high and low hepatic extraction ratio drugs.

? Self-test questions

1. The main determinants of the hepatic clearance of a low hepatic extraction ratio drug are:

   a) intrinsic clearance

   b) hepatic blood flow

   c) elimination rate

   d) protein binding

   e) dose

2. The main determinants of the hepatic clearance of a high hepatic extraction ratio drug are:
   a) intrinsic clearance
   b) hepatic blood flow
   c) elimination rate
   d) protein binding
   e) dose

3. The hepatic intrinsic clearance of a drug is determined by:
   a) the tightness of binding of the drug to plasma proteins
   b) the maximal rate at which it can be metabolised by the drug metabolising enzyme
   c) the blood flow to the liver
   d) the tightness of binding to the drug metabolising enzyme
   e) the hepatic extraction ratio

4. For drugs such as warfarin with a low hepatic extraction ratio, a twofold increase in the activity of the drug metabolising enzymes will approximately:
   a) halve hepatic extraction ratio
   b) double hepatic clearance
   c) double hepatic extraction ratio
   d) halve hepatic clearance
   e) double hepatic intrinsic clearance

5. For a high hepatic extraction ratio drug, a halving of hepatic blood flow will approximately:
   a) double hepatic extraction ratio
   b) halve hepatic clearance
   c) double hepatic intrinsic clearance
   d) double hepatic clearance
   e) halve hepatic intrinsic clearance

5

BIOAVAILABILITY AND FIRST-PASS CLEARANCE

Getting the definitions straight

As the terms absorption, first-pass clearance, bioavailability and bioequivalence are often used loosely, we should first make sure of the definitions.

- *Absorption:* is the extent to which intact drug is absorbed from the gut lumen into the portal circulation. This is expressed as the fraction of the dose which is absorbed from the gut, f_g.

  The factors affecting absorption are summarised in Table 5.1.

- *First-pass clearance:* is the extent to which a drug is removed by the liver during its first passage in the portal blood through the liver to the systemic circulation.

  This is also called first-pass metabolism or first-pass extraction. The fraction of drug which escapes first-pass clearance from the portal blood is expressed as f_H.

- *Bioavailability:* is the fraction of the dose which reaches the *systemic* circulation as intact drug. This is expressed as F.

  It is apparent that bioavailability will depend on both how well the drug is absorbed and how much escapes being removed by the liver before reaching the systemic circulation (Figure 5.1).

Bioavailability = fraction absorbed*fraction escaping first-pass clearance
$F = f_g * f_H$

Equation 5.1

where the fraction of drug escaping extraction by the liver is (1 – hepatic extraction ratio). The fact that it is (1 – hepatic extraction ratio) is important for bioavailability as will be seen below.

Table 5.1: Determinants of drug absorption from the gut

Dissolution
-   physico-chemical properties of drug
-   crystal size and form
-   excipients
-   special dosage forms (sustained release, enteric coated)
-   pH (stomach and small intestine)

Gastric emptying rate
-   stability of drug at acid pH
-   solution or solid dosage forms (liquids and small particles empty more quickly)
-   affected by: food; antacids; drugs (opiates, anticholinergics, meto-clopramide); disease (autonomic neuropathy)

Intestinal motility
-   dissolution of slowly soluble drugs (digoxin, sustained release for-mulations)
-   chemical degradation or metabolism by microflora

Drug interactions in the gut lumen
-   complexation (tetracyclines with divalent metal ions)
-   adsorption (anion exchange resins)
-   food interactions (many antibiotics)

Passage through the gut wall
-   physico-chemical characteristics of the drug (quaternary ammoni-um compounds)
-   metabolism by enzymes in the intestinal endothelium

- *Bioequivalence:* is a clinical definition referring to two for-mulations of a drug. Two formulations of the same drug are considered bioequivalent if the extents and rates of absorp-tion of drug from them are so similar that there is likely to be no clinically important difference between their effects, either therapeutic or adverse.

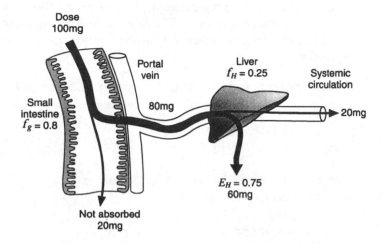

Figure 5.1: Factors affecting bioavailability

In this example, 80 mg of the original 100 mg dose is absorbed intact into the portal circulation (fraction absorbed is 0.8). The hepatic extraction ratio is 0.75, so that 60 mg is extracted in the first pass through the liver and 20 mg escapes extraction.

The bioavailability (see Equation 5.1) is $F = f_g*f_H$ which is $0.8*0.25 = 0.2$ (20%).

The clinical decision as to what would be a clinically important difference will vary from drug to drug. For example, small differences between formulations may be important for drugs such as digoxin which have low therapeutic ratios, or for drugs such as phenytoin which have non-linear kinetics. A larger difference may be tolerated for drugs such as amoxycillin which have high therapeutic ratios.

How is bioavailability measured?

Absolute bioavailability is measured against an intravenous reference dose (the bioavailability of an intravenous dose is 100% by definition). The usual method is to give a group of volunteers intravenous and oral doses of the drug on separate occasions. The areas under the plasma drug concentration versus time curves (AUC), after the two doses, are used to calculate the bioavailability of the oral formulation by simple proportion.

This is because:

$$AUC_{iv} = \frac{Dose_{iv}}{Clearance}$$

Equation 5.2

and

$$AUC_{oral} = \frac{F * Dose_{oral}}{Clearance}$$

Equation 5.3

so that

$$\frac{AUC_{oral}}{AUC_{iv}} = \frac{F * Dose_{oral}}{Dose_{iv}}$$

Equation 5.4

If the oral and intravenous doses are the same

$$F = \frac{AUC_{oral}}{AUC_{iv}}$$

Equation 5.5

For example, if the same intravenous and oral doses are given and AUC_{oral} is 50% of AUC_{iv}, the bioavailability of the oral formulation is 50%. This is illustrated in Figure 5.2. The fact that the bioavailability is only 50% might be due to incomplete absorption, first-pass clearance or a combination of these.

Other methods, which are used less frequently, include comparing the urinary recoveries of drug or metabolite after intravenous and oral doses, or measuring the steady state plasma drug concentrations during intravenous and oral dosing.

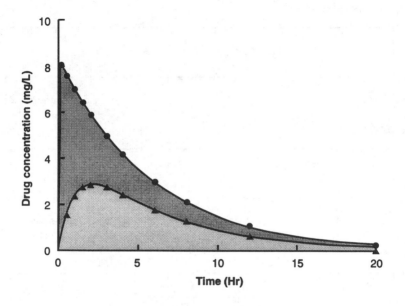

Figure 5.2: Plasma concentration time curves of equal intravenous and oral doses of a drug

The area under the curve for the oral formulation (AUC_{oral}) is 50% of the area under the curve for the intravenous dose (AUC_{iv}). The absolute bioavailability of the oral formulation is 0.5. The incomplete bioavailability could be due to poor absorption or first-pass clearance or a combination of these ($F = f_g*f_H$). The areas under the two curves are $AUC_{iv} = 48.1$ mg*hour/L and $AUC_{oral} = 24.05$ mg*hour/L.

The bioavailability of one oral formulation (the test formulation) is often assessed against a second oral (reference) formulation. This is referred to as measuring relative bioavailability, and is commonly done for new generic products where the reference formulation is the innovator's brand or the market leader formulation (brand) for that drug. It is called relative bioavailability as the absolute bioavailability of both formulations might be quite low due to poor absorption and/or first-pass clearance, and this would not be detected. This type of study provides a measure of the relative performance of two formulations in getting drug absorbed. The criterion used for the bioequivalence of two such formulations is usually that the ratio of their AUCs should be in the range 0.8 to 1.25.

$$relative\ bioavailability = \frac{AUC_{test}}{AUC_{reference}}$$

Equation 5.6

What determines first-pass clearance?

Let us now concentrate on first-pass clearance and, for the moment, assume that the entire dose is absorbed intact from the gut lumen into the portal circulation. The bioavailability then depends only on the fraction escaping first-pass hepatic extraction as the fraction absorbed into the portal circulation (f_g) is 1.0 (see Equation 5.1). Then:

$$bioavailability = (1 - hepatic\ extraction\ ratio)$$

Equation 5.7

The determinants of hepatic extraction ratio were considered in detail in Chapter 4. Let us take the same two limiting cases as previously, and look at the effects on bioavailability of increasing or decreasing the hepatic extraction ratio by changing the activity of the liver drug metabolising enzymes. Table 5.2 summarises these effects.

Low hepatic extraction ratio drugs

In the case of drugs such as theophylline which are poorly extracted by the liver, nearly all the dose gets through the liver first pass and bioavailability is essentially complete as long as they are well absorbed from the gut. Even doubling or halving the minor proportion extracted by the liver does not make any significant difference to bioavailability (see Table 5.2).

Table 5.2: Effects of increase or decrease in hepatic drug metabolising enzyme activity on bioavailability

Hepatic enzyme activity	% extracted first pass	Bioavailability (% escaping first-pass clearance)
Low extraction ratio drug		
Normal	2	98
Doubled (induced)	4	96
Halved (inhibited)	1	99
High extraction ratio drug		
Normal	90	10
Doubled (induced)	95	5
Halved (inhibited)	83	17

All the dose is assumed to be absorbed intact from the gut lumen. The low extraction ratio example is characteristic of theophylline which has a clearance (see Chapter 4) of about 1.8 L/hour. The high extraction ratio example is characteristic of verapamil which has a clearance of about 80 L/hour. Liver blood flow is normally around 90 L/hour.

High hepatic extraction ratio drugs

For drugs such as verapamil, which are efficiently extracted by the liver, most of the dose is extracted on the first pass through the liver so that only a minor proportion reaches the systemic circulation intact (Table 5.2). Inducing or inhibiting the metabolising enzymes has only a small effect on hepatic extraction ratio, and thus on *systemic* clearance (see previous chapter), **but has a major effect on the proportion *escaping* extraction which is (1 – hepatic extraction ratio), and thus has a major effect on bioavailability** (Table 5.2).

For these drugs, hepatic enzyme activity is a major determinant of first-pass metabolism and oral bioavailability, whereas hepatic blood flow is the major determinant of systemic clearance. Changes in hepatic blood flow do alter the first-pass clearance and bioavailability of high hepatic extraction ratio drugs. However, changes in hepatic blood flow also alter the systemic clearance of these drugs. The two effects are in opposite directions, about equal in magnitude and therefore cancel each other out. This is discussed further in Chapter 6.

Why is first-pass clearance important?

- *Variability in drug response.* As seen from Table 5.2, even small changes in the hepatic extraction ratio of drugs such as verapamil can cause large changes in bioavailability. Thus, the plasma concentrations of such drugs after oral administration are often more variable, both within and between individuals, than the plasma concentrations of drugs with close to complete bioavailability.

- *Relationship between oral and intravenous doses.* With the high extraction ratio drug in Table 5.2, only 10% of the oral dose reaches the systemic circulation as against, by definition, 100% of an intravenous dose. If there are no other complicating factors, the oral dose will therefore have to be 10 times the intravenous dose to achieve similar plasma concentrations and effects by the two routes of administration. For drugs with complete bioavailability, oral and intravenous doses are similar.

- *Alternative routes of administration.* Some drugs are so highly extracted by the liver that their oral bioavailability is negligible. Glyceryl trinitrate and ergotamine are examples, both having first-pass clearances of 99% or more and therefore oral bioavailabilities of less than 1% of the dose. Glyceryl trinitrate is administered by the sublingual route because the venous drainage from the mouth goes directly to the systemic circulation and first-pass clearance by the liver is avoided. Transdermal administration of glyceryl trinitrate achieves the same result and also provides a slow, sustained delivery of drug.

Part of the rectal circulation (about one-third) is systemic rather than portal, so rectal administration reduces first-pass clearance. However, absorption of drugs from the rectum is often erratic and incomplete.

Administration by inhalation can also be used for systemic delivery to avoid first-pass clearance of some drugs (for example, ergotamine). When drugs are used by inhalation for local effects on the lung, extensive first-pass clearance can be a protective mechanism against systemic effects of the drug which is swallowed (often as much as 90% of the inhaled dose) rather than passing to the lungs. Examples are the $beta_2$-adrenoreceptor agonist salbutamol and the inhaled corticosteroid beclomethasone.

- *Drug interactions.* As seen in Table 5.2, induction or inhibition of drug metabolising enzymes in the liver by other drugs or environmental agents such as cigarette smoke can cause large changes in the oral bioavailability of high, but not low, clearance drugs. An example of this effect is shown in Figure 5.3 (on following page).

- *Liver disease.* In chronic liver disease, a substantial part of the portal circulation does not perfuse functional liver cells due to the presence of intrahepatic functional shunts or extrahepatic anatomic shunts. If 50% of the portal blood does not perfuse functioning liver cells, then 50% of first-pass clearance will be avoided and bioavailability increased markedly. With the high extraction ratio drug in Table 5.2, bioavailability and effective dose would be increased from 10% to 55% (ie, 5.5-fold) in this situation. **Thus, high hepatic extraction drugs given to patients with liver disease are particularly liable to cause an increased incidence of adverse effects.**

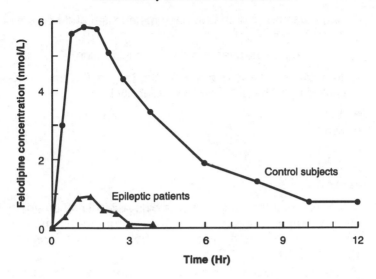

Figure 5.3: Effect on felodipine bioavailability due to a drug interaction with anticonvulsants

● healthy control subjects; ▲ epileptic patients on liver enzyme inducing anticonvulsants

The relative oral bioavailability in epileptic patients was reduced to 6.6% of that in healthy control subjects. As the usual absolute oral bioavailability of felodipine (compared to an intravenous dose) is about 15%, only about 1% of an oral dose would be absorbed intact in patients on enzyme-inducing anticonvulsants. In this study, 10 out of 12 control subjects, but none of the epileptic patients, experienced vasodilator effects. In four of the 10 epileptic patients, felodipine could not be detected in plasma.

Adapted with permission from *Lancet* 1988;2:481.

 Self-test questions

1. Bioavailability:
   a) is the extent to which a drug is absorbed from the gut
   b) is the fraction of the drug metabolised first pass by the liver
   c) is the fraction of the dose reaching the systemic circulation intact

    d) is a measure of both first-pass metabolism and absorption from the gut

    e) only refers to intravenous drug administration

2. A drug has a hepatic extraction ratio (E_H) of 0.6 and is 40% absorbed from the gut. The bioavailability is:

    a) 0.4

    b) 0.6

    c) 0.16

    d) 0.24

    e) 0.10

3. A new generic drug is tested in a bioavailability study against the innovator brand. The AUC_{oral} for the generic is 1200 mg*hour/L and that for the innovator brand is 1000 mg*hour/L.

    a) the relative bioavailability of the generic formulation compared to the innovator brand is 1.2

    b) the absolute bioavailability of the innovator brand is 1.0

    c) the generic formulation would usually be regarded as bioequivalent to the innovator brand

    d) the absolute bioavailability of the innovator brand is 0.83

    e) the generic brand is better than the innovator brand

4. For low hepatic extraction ratio drugs which are completely absorbed, doubling the hepatic extraction ratio:

    a) doubles the bioavailability

    b) makes little difference to the bioavailability

    c) halves the bioavailability

    d) reduces the bioavailability by 40%

    e) increases the bioavailability by 40%

5. Which of the following routes of administration completely avoid first-pass clearance?

    a) buccal

    b) sublingual

    c) rectal

    d) oral

    e) transdermal

6

PREDICTING DRUG INTERACTIONS AND THE EFFECTS OF DISEASE STATES FOR METABOLISED DRUGS

For drugs which are cleared mainly by metabolism, we looked in Chapter 4 at the physiological factors which determine systemic clearance, and in Chapter 5 at factors which determine first-pass clearance. Drugs given orally are subject to both first-pass clearance and systemic clearance. We now have to put these together and look at the physiological processes determining steady state concentration (C_{ss}) of various types of drugs when they are given either orally or intravenously (systemically). For the moment, we will continue to assume that the drug is totally metabolised and completely absorbed from the gut ($f_g = 1.0$), and will then go on to see how knowledge of a few very simple pharmacokinetic parameters can allow rather wide-ranging predictions of how a drug will behave in practice.

What determines steady state drug concentrations during chronic dosing?

The first point to note is that it is generally the unbound drug (drug not bound to plasma proteins or blood cells — see Chapter 8) which interacts with receptors and produces drug effects. We will therefore have to look at the physiological factors determining both unbound and total drug concentrations at steady state during continuous dosing. Once again, the two limiting examples of high and low hepatic clearance drugs will be considered. Table 6.1 summarises the factors involved.

Table 6.1: Physiological parameters determining steady state concentrations of highly metabolised drugs during chronic dosing

Type of drug and examples	Determinants of steady state blood concentration	
	Unbound concentration	*Total concentration*
Oral administration		
Low hepatic extraction ratio	Intrinsic clearance	Intrinsic clearance and fraction unbound
High hepatic extraction ratio	Intrinsic clearance	Intrinsic clearance and fraction unbound
Intravenous administration		
Low hepatic extraction ratio	Intrinsic clearance	Intrinsic clearance and fraction unbound
High hepatic extraction ratio	Hepatic blood flow and fraction unbound	Hepatic blood flow

For *orally* administered drugs, a combination of factors determining first-pass clearance and systemic clearance (of the drug escaping first-pass extraction) are involved. For *intravenously* administered drugs, only systemic clearance is important.

Fortunately, when all the equations are solved, the situation turns out to be very simple. In all circumstances except one, the sole determinant of steady state unbound drug concentrations is the activity of the drug-metabolising enzymes in the liver (intrinsic clearance). This applies to low clearance drugs given either orally or intravenously (systemic clearance is important here — see Chapter 4) and to high clearance drugs given orally (first-pass clearance is of major importance here — see Chapter 5). It follows that circumstances which alter the drug-metabolising enzymes, such as co-administration of inducers or inhibitors, will alter steady state drug concentrations and effects of all metabolised drugs given orally. Circumstances which alter liver blood flow, such as cardiac failure, will usually be of less importance unless this also affects the activity of the drug-metabolising enzymes.

Changes in hepatic blood flow do not affect the steady state concentrations of high hepatic extraction ratio drugs given orally. This is because, as noted in Chapter 5, effects of changes in hepatic blood flow on first-pass clearance and systemic clearance cancel each other out. In contrast, changes in intrinsic clearance do affect steady state concentrations of high extraction ratio drugs given orally — the change produced in first-pass clearance is not compensated in this case by a change in systemic clearance which is determined by hepatic blood flow.

It will be apparent from Table 6.1 that *total* but not *unbound* drug concentrations are affected by protein binding. The importance of protein binding — or perhaps the lack of importance — is considered in Chapter 8.

For those relatively few instances where high clearance drugs are given systemically for long enough to reach steady state, hepatic blood flow and protein binding are the determinants of unbound drug concentrations. With these drugs, virtually all the drug delivered to the liver is extracted during a single pass through the liver, so the rate of delivery (hepatic blood flow) becomes the main factor. Protein binding is important because the higher the binding, the more drug is 'held' in the blood for presentation to and extraction by the liver. Examples of such high hepatic extraction ratio drugs are lignocaine given intravenously for cardiac arrhythmias, and morphine given systemically (intravenous or intramuscular dosing) for pain. Factors which alter liver blood flow, such as cardiac failure, exert major effects on the steady state concentrations of such drugs.

How to determine the relative importance of metabolism and renal excretion

So far we have been assuming that the drug is nearly completely metabolised. In fact, all drugs are partly metabolised and partly excreted unchanged by the kidney. The usual way to determine the relative importance of the two elimination mechanisms for a particular drug is to give a dose of the drug, collect all the urine, measure how much drug comes out unchanged (the rest is metabolised) and express this as a fraction of the dose given. This is *the fraction excreted unchanged (f_e),* which can vary from close to 0 (nearly all the drug is metabolised, for example, propranolol, morphine, tolbutamide, theophylline) to close to 1 (nearly all the drug is excreted unchanged, for example, penicillin, amoxycillin, gentamicin, digoxin). It is apparent that *the fraction of the dose which is metabolised* is (1 − fraction excreted unchanged).

Clearances are additive — calculating hepatic and renal clearances

The total body clearance is the sum of all the individual clearance processes occurring. As these are usually mainly renal clearance of unchanged drug and hepatic clearance by metabolism:

$$total\ clearance\ =\ renal\ clearance\ +\ hepatic\ clearance$$

Equation 6.1

The fraction of drug excreted unchanged is then the fraction which renal clearance represents of total clearance:

$$fraction\ excreted\ unchanged\ =\ \frac{renal\ clearance}{total\ clearance}$$

Equation 6.2

and the fraction metabolised is:

$$fraction\ metabolised\ =\ \frac{hepatic\ clearance}{total\ clearance}$$

Equation 6.3

or

$$fraction\ metabolised = \frac{total\ clearance\ -\ renal\ clearance}{total\ clearance}$$

Equation 6.4

It follows from these relationships that knowing the total clearance and the fraction excreted unchanged, renal clearance can be calculated from Equation 6.2, hepatic clearance from Equation 6.1, and the fraction metabolised from Equation 6.4 or as (1 – fraction excreted unchanged).

Also, the hepatic extraction ratio (E_H — see Chapter 4) can be calculated from the hepatic clearance (CL_H) and hepatic blood flow (Q_H) as:

$$hepatic\ extraction\ ratio = \frac{hepatic\ clearance}{hepatic\ blood\ flow}$$

$$E_H = \frac{CL_H}{Q_H}$$

Equation 6.5

and the maximum oral bioavailability if the drug was totally absorbed from the gut into the portal circulation can then be calculated as:

$$F = f_g * f_H \quad where\ f_g = 1.0\ and\ f_H = (1 - E_H)$$

Equation 6.6

Predicting everything about a drug from a few simple pharmacokinetic parameters

Because pharmacokinetics is now described in terms of physiological processes, it is possible to predict how changes in these processes — due, for example, to drug interactions or disease states — will affect the handling of a drug by the body. This is illustrated in Table 6.2 for three different types of drugs. We will look at how it works for Drug A and you can complete the Table for Drugs B and C.

Table 6.2: Predicting how drugs will behave pharmacokinetically in various situations

Known parameters	Drug A	Drug B	Drug C
Total clearance (L/hour)	80	3	7
Volume of distribution (L)	500	25	420
Fraction excreted unchanged	0.1	0.1	0.8
Liver blood flow (L/hour)	90	90	90
Predicted			
Renal clearance (L/hour)	8		
Hepatic clearance (L/hour)	72		
Hepatic extraction ratio	0.8		
Maximum oral bioavailability (%)	20		
Affected by induction/inhibition of liver enzymes when given orally	Yes		
Affected by liver blood flow (eg cardiac failure) when given intravenously	Yes		
Decrease dose in liver disease	Yes		
Decrease dose in renal failure	No		
Half-life (hour) (see Equation 3.3)	4		
Likely dosing schedule (times per day)	6		
Time to reach steady state (hour)	20		

The completed information for Drug B and Drug C can be found on p 52.

If total body clearance, volume of distribution and the fraction excreted unchanged are known, the rest can be calculated or predicted as follows:

- The fraction of the dose of Drug A which is metabolised $(1 - f_e)$ is 0.9 $(1 - 0.1)$ and from Equation 6.3 the hepatic clearance is therefore 72 L/hour $(0.9*80)$. As liver blood flow is around 90 L/hour, the hepatic extraction ratio is 0.8 $(72 \div 90)$ (see Equation 6.5 above and also Chapter 4). The fraction escaping first-pass clearance, f_H, is therefore 0.2 $(1 - 0.8)$, so that the *maximum* oral bioavailability will be 20% ($F = f_g*f_H$). It might be even less if the drug is also poorly absorbed from the gut into the portal circulation (see Chapter 5).

- The drug has a relatively high hepatic extraction ratio (0.8), so from Table 6.1 we can see the steady state drug concentration will be determined mainly by hepatic enzyme activity when given orally and by liver blood flow when given systemically. There will be decreases in both first-pass clearance (increased oral bioavailability) and systemic clearance in liver disease so dose reduction will be mandatory. Only 10% is renally cleared (fraction excreted unchanged is 0.1) so dose reduction will not be necessary in renal failure unless there are active metabolites which are mainly renally cleared.

- From the volume of distribution and the clearance, the half-life is calculated as 4 hours (see Chapter 3). Dosing will thus need to be 4–6 times a day unless a sustained release form is available. Steady state will be reached after about one day of treatment (3–5 half-lives — see Chapter 3).

Put briefly, when given pharmacokinetic information about a drug, as in product information, it is only necessary to ask the following questions to predict reasonably well what clinical situations are likely to require care or possible dose alterations due to a potential for changed pharmacokinetics.

- Is it mainly metabolised or mainly renally excreted?
- If metabolised, does it have high or low hepatic clearance?
- What is the half-life?
- Are there complicating factors such as active metabolites?

In the next chapter, we will see how similar predictions can be made for renally excreted drugs based on a knowledge of the processes by which they are excreted.

Answers to Table 6.2 (p 50)

Known parameters	Drug B	Drug C
Total clearance (L/hour)	3	7
Volume of distribution (L)	25	420
Fraction excreted unchanged	0.1	0.8
Liver blood flow (L/hour)	90	90
Predicted		
Renal clearance (L/hour)	0.3	5.6
Hepatic clearance (L/hour)	2.7	1.4
Hepatic extraction ratio	0.03	0.015
Maximum oral bioavailability (%)	97	98.5
Affected by induction/inhibition of liver enzymes when given orally	Yes	No
Affected by liver blood flow (eg cardiac failure) when given intravenously	No	No
Decrease dose in liver disease	Yes	No
Decrease dose in renal failure	No	Yes
Half-life (hour) (see Equation 3.3)	6	40
Likely dosing schedule (times per day)	4	1
Time to reach steady state (hour)	30	200

Drug A has the characteristics of propranolol, pethidine, verapamil

Drug B has the characteristics of theophylline, tolbutamide

Drug C has the characteristics of digoxin

? Self-test questions

1. The determinants of the total (bound and unbound) steady state concentration of a high hepatic extraction ratio drug during oral dosing are:
   a) hepatic blood flow
   b) hepatic enzyme activity
   c) renal blood flow
   d) fraction unbound in plasma
   e) cardiac output

2. The determinants of the unbound steady state concentration of a low hepatic extraction ratio metabolised drug during oral dosing are:
   a) hepatic intrinsic clearance
   b) renal intrinsic clearance
   c) fraction unbound in plasma
   d) hepatic blood flow
   e) glomerular filtration rate

3. The determinants of the unbound steady state concentration of a high hepatic extraction ratio drug during intravenous dosing are:
   a) fraction unbound in plasma
   b) hepatic intrinsic clearance
   c) hepatic drug metabolising enzyme activity
   d) hepatic blood flow
   e) renal clearance

4. A drug has a hepatic clearance of 72 L/hour and liver blood flow is 90 L/hour. Its maximum oral bioavailability is likely to be:
   a) 100%
   b) 80%
   c) 50%
   d) 20%
   e) 10%

5. A drug has a fraction excreted unchanged (f_e) of 0.1 and a total body clearance (CL) of 50 L/hour. Liver blood flow is 90 L/hour. Its maximum oral bioavailability is likely to be:

   a) 90%

   b) 75%

   c) 50%

   d) 25%

   e) 10%

7

CLEARANCE OF DRUGS BY THE KIDNEYS

So far we have considered drug clearance as though it is all due to liver metabolism. In Chapter 6, the concept of 'fraction excreted unchanged' was introduced to determine the relative importance of elimination by metabolism and elimination (excretion) unchanged by the kidneys. Many drugs have low metabolic clearance relative to their renal clearance, so that renal clearance becomes the dominant factor in their handling by the body.

How are drugs cleared by the kidneys?

Renal drug clearance is the net result of three different processes as shown in Figure 7.1. Drug is cleared from the blood into the urine by filtration at the glomerulus and active secretion in the proximal tubule, and is passively reabsorbed from the urine back into the blood all along the renal tubule.

> *renal clearance = filtration + secretion − reabsorption*

Equation 7.1

We will now consider each of these processes separately.

Glomerular filtration

As blood passes through the glomerulus (1200 mL/minute), about 10% is filtered as plasma water into the renal tubule (that is, glomerular filtration rate (GFR) is about 120 mL/minute), and drug in plasma water (unbound drug) goes with it. Drug bound to plasma proteins is not filtered. Thus, the renal clearance by glomerular filtration (CL_{GF}) is:

$$CL_{GF} = fu*GFR$$

Equation 7.2

where fu is the fraction of drug unbound in plasma.

If nothing further happens to the drug — that is, it is neither secreted nor reabsorbed — then this will be its net renal clearance. Creatinine and inulin are not bound to plasma proteins (fraction unbound is 1), are not secreted and are not reabsorbed. This allows their renal clearances to be used as measures of GFR.

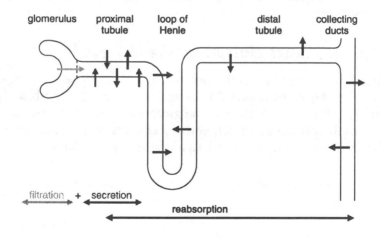

Figure 7.1: Renal drug elimination

Renal drug clearance is the net result of filtration clearance (at the glomerulus) plus clearance by active secretion (in the proximal tubule) minus reabsorption which occurs all along the renal tubule.

Active tubular secretion

The proximal tubule contains at least two active transport mechanisms (pumps) to move drug from the blood into the renal tubule. This component of renal clearance, secretion clearance, is designated as CL_S. The secretion mechanisms are so active with some drugs that even bound drug can be stripped off plasma proteins in one pass of the blood through the kidney. This is a similar situation to that of high hepatic extraction ratio drugs in the liver (see Chapter 4). Most secreted drugs, however, have low intrinsic clearance by secretion and only unbound drug is secreted. The clearance by secretion then becomes $fu*CL_S$.

There are two major active transport systems: one for drugs which are weak acids (negatively charged) and one for drugs which are weak bases (positively charged). There are two important consequences arising from the active secretion mechanisms.

- *Competitive drug interactions*. Competition for the active transport systems can occur, leading to desirable or undesirable drug interactions. Weak acids compete with weak acids and weak bases with weak bases. For example, penicillin and probenecid are both substrates for the acid pump, so probenecid is used to compete with penicillin to reduce its renal clearance and intensify and prolong its action. Cimetidine and procainamide are basic drugs which compete with each other for the base secretion mechanism and thus reduce each other's renal clearance and increase steady state drug concentrations.

- *Saturable kinetics*. The active processes are saturable so that renal clearance can become non-linear at high doses (see Chapter 9).

Para-aminohippuric acid (PAH) is so actively secreted by the acid secretion system that essentially all the PAH is removed from the renal blood in one pass through the kidney. As PAH is not reabsorbed in the renal tubule, its clearance is a measure of renal blood flow. In a similar fashion to hepatic clearance (see Chapter 4), renal drug clearance cannot be greater than renal blood flow.

Passive tubular reabsorption

Most of the 120 mL/minute of plasma water filtered at the glomerulus is reabsorbed during its passage through the renal tubule, so that only about 1–2 mL/minute finally appears as urine. If the drug filtered in the plasma water was neither secreted nor reabsorbed, it would therefore be concentrated in urine to about 100 times the unbound concentration in plasma. However, as plasma water is reabsorbed, a concentration gradient is established between drug in the tubular fluid and unbound drug in the blood. If the drug is able to pass through the membranes of the tubular cell, it moves down this concentration gradient and is reabsorbed from the tubular fluid back into the blood. What determines if this occurs? The first factor is the magnitude of the concentration gradient, which obviously depends on the extent of water reabsorption. If the urine is dilute (urine flow is high, less of the filtered water is being reabsorbed), the concentration gradient is less, and less drug is reabsorbed. *For drugs which are reabsorbed, renal clearance varies with urine flow rate.* The higher the flow, the greater the clearance. An example of this (the renal clearance of caffeine) is shown in Figure 7.2.

The second factor is the ease with which the drug can move through the membranes of the tubule cells. Only non-ionised drugs can pass through the lipid membrane and the ease with which this occurs depends on the lipid solubility of the non-ionised drug. The extent to which the drug is non-ionised depends on the pH of the urine and the pK_a of the drug. *For drugs which are lipid soluble enough to be reabsorbed, and can ionise to an anion or a cation, renal clearance varies with urine pH.*

Renal clearance

We can now assemble the three components, glomerular filtration, active tubular secretion and passive tubular reabsorption, to derive an expression for renal clearance.

$$CL_R = fu \, (GFR + CL_S) \, (1 - FR)$$

Equation 7.3

Renal clearance is the sum of glomerular filtration clearance (fu*GFR) and secretion clearance (fu*CL$_S$) multiplied by the fraction of drug that escapes reabsorption from the renal tubule (1 − FR).

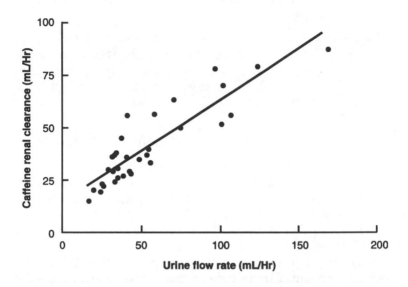

Figure 7.2: Effect of urine flow rate on caffeine renal clearance

Caffeine is reabsorbed essentially to equilibrium with unbound caffeine in blood. Renal caffeine clearance is directly proportional to urine flow rate but is low so that only 1–2% is excreted unchanged, with metabolism being the major elimination mechanism.

How to tell if a drug is secreted or reabsorbed

All drugs are filtered so there is a baseline renal clearance of fu*GFR. From Equation 7.3, if actual renal drug clearance is *greater* than fu*GFR, the drug must be secreted — it *may* also be reabsorbed, but to a lesser extent than it is secreted. If actual renal clearance is *less* than fu*GFR, it must be reabsorbed — it *may* also be secreted, but to a lesser extent than it is reabsorbed.

To check for secretion or reabsorption, the following can be done.

- If the drug is a weak acid or a weak base, a known competitor, for example, probenecid (acid) or cimetidine (base), can be given. If renal clearance is reduced, the drug is likely to be secreted.

- The effect of changing urine flow rate and/or pH can be investigated. If renal drug clearance changes when urine flow rate or pH changes, it is likely that the drug is reabsorbed. For example, if the urine is made more alkaline the excretion of acidic drugs will be increased.

Prediction of disease and drug interaction effects

Table 7.1 shows how the basic pharmacokinetic parameters of a drug can be used to make predictions about renal elimination mechanisms and renal drug interactions. The answers are shown for ampicillin and you should fill in the table for gentamicin and procainamide. For ampicillin, renal clearance is about 10 L/hour (fraction eliminated unchanged * clearance) (f_e*CL) which is substantially greater than fu*GFR (5.6 L/hour). This means that ampicillin must be secreted and may or may not be reabsorbed in the renal tubule. As it is an acidic drug which is secreted, other acidic drugs will compete for the 'acid pump' and reduce its clearance (for example, probenecid). This will not apply to basic drugs such as cimetidine. Urine flow rate and/or pH will only affect renal clearance if it is in fact reabsorbed to some extent. Renal clearance will be reduced proportionately with creatinine clearance in renal dysfunction (see below), so total plasma clearance will be reduced to 20% of normal in the complete absence of renal function (f_e is 0.8, so renal clearance is 80% of total plasma clearance). Dose adjustment may not be necessary as the penicillins have high therapeutic indices (margins of safety).

Table 7.1: Prediction of renal excretion mechanisms and interactions

	Ampicillin	Gentamicin	Procainamide
Known parameters			
Clearance (L/hour)	13	6	25
Volume of distribution (L)	20	20	130
Fraction eliminated unchanged (f_e)	0.8	1	0.6
Fraction unbound in plasma (fu)	0.8	1	0.85
Acid or base	acid	base	base
Predicted			
Renal clearance (f_e*CL) (L/hour)	10		
fu*GFR (L/hour)*	5.6		
Secreted	yes		
Reabsorbed	possible		
Interact with: probenecid	yes		
cimetidine	no		
Affected by urine flow rate/pH	possible		
Adjust dose in renal failure	yes/no		

* for this exercise, assume GFR is 7 L/hour

The completed information for gentamicin and procainamide can be found on p 63.

Dose adjustment in renal dysfunction

No matter what the elimination mechanism, the renal clearance of drugs is reduced in proportion with the reduction in creatinine clearance (glomerular filtration rate). This is known as the intact tubule hypothesis. The kidney behaves as though the total number of renal tubules is reduced, with those remaining acting normally.

Therefore, creatinine clearance provides a simple guide to the reduction of dose rate in renal dysfunction. As *serum* creatinine is determined by both its rate of production from muscle and its rate of elimination, corrections have to be applied for gender, weight and age to enable its use as an index of creatinine clearance.[1] The following guidelines apply to the adjustment of dose in renal failure.

- Adjustment is usually only necessary when a drug is more than 50% cleared by renal elimination (f_e >0.5) and renal function is reduced to half of normal or less.

- Dose *rate* is reduced proportionately to the reduction in creatinine clearance with allowance for the fraction of drug eliminated unchanged. For example, if the fraction of drug eliminated unchanged is 0.5 and creatinine clearance is reduced to 10% of normal, dose rate should be reduced to 55% of normal.[2] The dose rate can be reduced either by reduction in the size of each dose, or by lengthening the dosage interval, or both. For example, the dose *size* of digoxin is usually reduced with the doses continuing to be given once per day, which is convenient. By contrast, the dose *interval* for gentamicin is usually increased so that each dose is large enough to give adequate peak concentrations, but trough concentrations do not accumulate above safe levels.

Other questions which need to be asked in deciding whether to reduce dose in renal failure are:

- Does the drug have a narrow therapeutic index and concentration related toxicity? Penicillin is almost entirely

---

1.   *creatinine clearance* = $\dfrac{(140 - age)(weight\ in\ kg)}{814* serum\ creatinine\ (mmol/L)}$

Multiply by 0.85 for females

2.   This is calculated as follows:

Non-renal clearance is unchanged (50% of normal total clearance); renal clearance is reduced from 50% to 5% of normal total clearance; total clearance is therefore reduced to 50 + 5 = 55% of normal total clearance.

eliminated unchanged, but the dose is usually not altered in renal failure as the therapeutic index is high. This contrasts with gentamicin and digoxin which have narrow therapeutic indices.

- Does the drug have active metabolites which are renally eliminated (for example, metabolites of procainamide, allopurinol), or metabolites such as ester glucuronides which can be recycled to the parent drug when their renal elimination is reduced (for example, clofibrate)?

As with hepatic drug clearance, an understanding of the physiological mechanisms determining renal drug elimination allows general predictions about problems which might occur due to drug interactions or disturbed renal physiology.

Answers to Table 7.1 (p 61)

	Gentamicin	Procainamide
Known parameters		
Clearance (L/hour)	6	25
Volume of distribution (L)	20	130
Fraction eliminated unchanged (f_e)	1	0.6
Fraction unbound in plasma (fu)	1	0.85
Acid or base	base	base
Predicted		
Renal clearance (f_e*CL) (L/hour)	6	15
fu*GFR (L/hour)	7	6
Secreted	possible	yes
Reabsorbed	yes	possible
Interact with: probenecid	no	no
cimetidine	possible	yes
Affected by urine flow rate/pH	yes	possible
Adjust dose in renal failure	yes	yes

? Self-test questions

1. With respect to the renal clearance of drugs by glomerular filtration:
   a) glomerular filtration rate is about 40% of renal blood flow
   b) only unbound drug is filtered
   c) drug clearance by glomerular filtration is equal to glomerular filtration rate
   d) creatinine clearance is equal to drug clearance
   e) both bound and unbound drug can be filtered

2. The proportion of drug reabsorbed from the renal tubule depends on:
   a) the glomerular filtration rate
   b) the urine flow rate
   c) the extent of drug secretion into the renal tubule
   d) the lipophilicity of the non-ionised drug
   e) the urine pH

3. If a drug has a fraction unbound in plasma of 0.1 and a renal clearance of 20 L/hour, it is:
   a) possibly secreted into the renal tubule
   b) filtered at the glomerulus
   c) definitely secreted into the renal tubule
   d) possibly subject to tubular reabsorption
   e) definitely subject to tubular reabsorption

4. If a drug has a fraction unbound in plasma of 0.8 and a renal clearance of 2 L/hour, it:
   a) is possibly subject to tubular reabsorption
   b) has a clearance by glomerular filtration of 5.6 L/hour
   c) is definitely secreted
   d) is possibly secreted
   e) is definitely subject to tubular reabsorption

5. The renal clearance of a liphophilic drug which is a weak acid with a pK_a of 5.0 is likely to be:

a) reduced by cimetidine
b) reduced by probenecid
c) increased by acidifying the urine
d) increased by alkalinising the urine
e) increased by an increase in urine flow rate

8

DRUG PROTEIN BINDING

What is protein binding?

Drug protein binding is the reversible interaction of drugs with proteins in plasma. Drugs can also bind reversibly to red blood cell and tissue membranes and other blood and tissue constituents. Protein binding can be represented as:

$$free\ drug + free\ protein \rightleftharpoons drug\text{--}protein\ complex$$

Equation 8.1

It is important to remember that the process is reversible and that the rates of drug binding and release are very fast, occurring in the millisecond range. This means that if, for example, liver cells very efficiently extract free drug from the blood, the drug–protein complex can rapidly dissociate and drug initially bound to protein can be extracted in one pass through the liver (see Chapter 4).

What are the binding proteins in plasma?

The major drug binding proteins in plasma are:
- albumin
- alpha$_1$-acid glycoprotein
- lipoproteins

Albumin and alpha$_1$-acid glycoprotein have structurally selective binding sites for drugs, in the same way that the active sites of enzymes are structurally selective for substrates.

Each albumin molecule has at least six distinct binding sites for drugs and endogenous compounds. Two of these very tightly and specifically bind long chain fatty acids. There is another site which selectively binds bilirubin. There are two major drug binding sites called site I and site II which mainly bind acidic drugs. Site I binds drugs such as warfarin and phenylbutazone, whereas site II binds drugs such as diazepam and ibuprofen. Drugs which bind at the same site can be predicted to displace each other competitively when administered together.

Alpha$_1$-acid glycoprotein is an acute phase reactant which has one binding site selective for basic drugs such as disopyramide and lignocaine.

'Binding' of drugs to lipoproteins and red cell and other membranes is more a dissolving of the drugs in the lipids of the membrane rather than a true binding reaction. Very lipid soluble drugs partition preferentially into the membrane lipids rather than the plasma water. Some drugs bind strongly to particular tissue components such as DNA (for example, some anticancer drugs and quinacrine) and melanin-rich tissues (for example, chloroquine, amiodarone).

What determines extent of binding to plasma proteins?

The binding of a drug to a protein binding site is a saturable process governed by the same mass action expression that describes the interaction of a substrate with an enzyme binding site. The extent to which a drug is bound in plasma or blood is usually expressed as the fraction unbound (fu).

$$fraction\ unbound\ (fu)\ =\ \frac{unbound\ drug\ concentration}{total\ drug\ concentration}$$

Equation 8.2

The tighter the binding, the lower is the fraction unbound. The distinction between *fraction* unbound and unbound *concentration* is important as we shall see below. The fraction unbound of a drug is determined by:

- the affinity of the drug for the protein
- the concentration of the binding protein
- the concentration of drug relative to that of the binding protein.

In most cases, drug concentrations at therapeutic doses are well below those of the binding protein and the fraction unbound is constant across the therapeutic range of drug concentration. However, the concentration of alpha$_1$-acid glycoprotein is relatively low, and saturation of the binding sites can occur in the therapeutic range. An example is disopyramide where the unbound concentration increases linearly with dose, but there is a less than proportionate increase in total concentration as saturation occurs causing fraction unbound to increase. Albumin concentrations are high, and saturation rarely occurs with drugs binding to this protein. An exception is salicylate which has high therapeutic concentrations.

The concentration of albumin is decreased in liver disease and renal disease resulting in decreased drug binding. Alpha$_1$-acid glycoprotein is an acute phase reactant and concentrations increase in rheumatoid arthritis and post-myocardial infarction resulting in increased drug binding.

The binding affinity can be changed due to competition from endogenous compounds such as fatty acids, or from other drugs competing for the same protein binding sites.

Are protein binding drug interactions important?

Much has been made of the significance of protein binding interactions based on 'test-tube' experiments. For example, warfarin is about 99% bound and 1% unbound (fu = 0.01). If a competing drug reduces the binding from 99% to 98%, the *in vitro* unbound fraction rises from 0.01 to 0.02, a twofold increase. If nothing else happened, this would represent a twofold increase in the active unbound concentration.

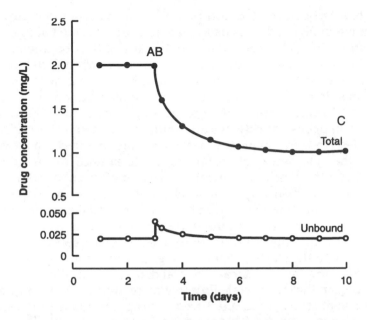

Figure 8.1: Sequence of events following displacement of a highly protein bound drug

Initially, the total concentration is 2 mg/L and the unbound concentration 0.02 mg/L, giving a fraction unbound of 0.01. Displacement occurs at A with addition of a displacing drug which is then continuously present. The fraction unbound increases to 0.02 and the unbound concentration doubles to 0.04 mg/L with no change in total concentration.

At B, redistribution occurs over minutes to hours resulting in decreases in both total and unbound concentrations. The clearance of unbound drug is not changed so the unbound concentration (C_{uss} = dose rate/CL_{int}) falls back to the initial value over 3–5 half-lives (half-life is 24 hours in this case).

At C, the final situation in the presence of displacing drug, total concentration is reduced by 50% to 1 mg/L, unbound concentration is the same as initially at 0.02 mg/L and fraction unbound is increased from 0.01 to 0.02. There is no change in drug effect. The example is based on warfarin displacement interactions.

In vivo, however, two compensating mechanisms operate as shown in Figure 8.1. As described in Chapter 2, the volume of distribution (V) is dependent on the ratio of fraction unbound in blood and tissues (fu/fu$_T$). If the fraction unbound in blood increases because of competitive displacement without a change in tissue binding, the volume of distribution increases as the displaced drug 'spreads out' and is bound in the tissues. This happens quickly within minutes to hours. Secondly, as described in Chapters 4 and 6, fraction unbound is a factor in the clearance of total drug (clearance = fraction unbound*intrinsic clearance), but clearance of unbound drug is determined only by intrinsic clearance and does not depend on protein binding. Therefore, when fraction unbound increases due to displacement, drug is eliminated more rapidly until the unbound (active) steady state concentration returns to the starting point. The end result is an increase in *unbound fraction*, a decrease in total drug concentration, but no change in the steady state *unbound concentration*. Total concentration at steady state is reduced in proportion to the increase in fraction unbound. This takes 3–5 half-lives to occur. In general, the only situation where unbound drug concentration at steady state is dependent on the degree of protein binding is that of high hepatic clearance drugs given intravenously (for example, lignocaine: see Chapters 4 and 6).

In nearly all cases where a clinically important protein binding interaction has been postulated, other mechanisms, such as concurrent inhibition of drug metabolism, have been shown to be the *in vivo* cause of the increase in drug effect. This is why it is so important in studies of drug interactions to measure *both* total and unbound drug in determining the mechanism(s). *Except in very rare circumstances, protein binding displacement in vivo does not result in increased drug effect.*

Protein binding and therapeutic drug monitoring

Drug assays for therapeutic drug monitoring nearly always measure total drug. As it is the unbound drug which is active, a false impression can be gained if the fraction unbound is changed substantially. This is illustrated in Table 8.1 for phenytoin. Phenytoin binding to albumin is reduced particularly in renal failure patients, but also in some other situations such as liver disease or the presence of competing drugs. In such cases, total concentration measurements are misleading and control of therapy needs to be based on measurement of unbound phenytoin concentration. Such measurements are available in specialised centres, but are expensive and currently are carried out only in special circumstances such as those mentioned above.

Table 8.1: Protein binding and the therapeutic range of phenytoin

Patient	fu	Therapeutic range based on total drug mg/L	Therapeutic range based on unbound drug mg/L
Normal	0.1	10–20	1–2
Renal failure	0.2	5–10	1–2

Phenytoin fraction unbound averages 0.1 in normal patients, but increases up to twofold in renal failure patients (GFR < 20 mL/minute) due to low albumin concentration and accumulation of competing endogenous compounds.

Summary

Protein binding is important in determining the cause of changes in total clearance due to drug interactions and in interpreting results of therapeutic monitoring of some drugs. In general, changes in protein binding *do not* cause clinically important drug interactions.

❓ Self-test questions

1. The fraction of a drug unbound in plasma is:
   a) usually not affected by the drug concentration
   b) independent of the concentration of binding protein
   c) dependent on the affinity of the drug for the binding protein
   d) usually increased as drug concentration increases
   e) usually decreased as drug concentration increases

2. With respect to the binding of drugs to plasma proteins:
   a) alpha$_1$-acid glycoprotein binds mainly basic drugs
   b) albumin has one binding site for drugs
   c) alpha$_1$-acid glycoprotein has one binding site for drugs
   d) lipoproteins bind drugs in a structurally specific manner
   e) albumin binds mainly acidic drugs

3. Warfarin normally has an unbound fraction in plasma of 0.01. If this was increased to 0.02 by displacement by a competing drug during chronic dosing:
   a) the unbound concentration at steady state would increase
   b) the unbound fraction at steady state would increase
   c) the volume of distribution would decrease
   d) warfarin toxicity would be likely
   e) clotting factor synthesis rate would not be altered

4. In the situation described in question 3:
   a) total warfarin clearance would be doubled
   b) unbound warfarin clearance would not change
   c) total steady state warfarin concentration would double
   d) total warfarin clearance would be halved
   e) unbound warfarin clearance would be halved

5. The usual therapeutic concentration range for phenytoin in terms of total drug is 10–20 mg/L. The unbound fraction of phenytoin in renal failure patients is increased from 0.1 to 0.2. With respect to the interpretation of the therapeutic drug monitoring of phenytoin in renal failure patients:

a) the therapeutic range in terms of total drug should be increased to 20–40 mg/L

b) the therapeutic range in terms of total drug should be reduced to 1–2 mg/L

c) the therapeutic range in terms of unbound drug should not be changed

d) the therapeutic range in terms of unbound drug should be doubled

e) the therapeutic range in terms of total drug should be reduced to 5–10 mg/L

9

NON-LINEAR PHARMACOKINETICS

What is meant by non-linear pharmacokinetics?

When the dose of a drug is increased, we expect that the concentration at steady state (C_{ss}) will increase proportionately; that is, if the dose rate is increased or decreased say twofold, the plasma drug concentration will also increase or decrease twofold. However, for some drugs, the plasma drug concentration changes either more or less than would be expected from a change in dose rate. This is known as non-linear pharmacokinetic behaviour and can cause problems when adjusting doses.

What causes non-linear pharmacokinetic behaviour?

In Chapter 1 it was shown that the steady state blood concentration (C_{ss}) is a function of the dose rate, the bioavailability and the clearance of the drug.

$$C_{ss} = \frac{F * dose\ rate}{clearance}$$

Equation 9.1

where F is the bioavailability.

For low hepatic extraction ratio drugs, clearance (CL) is determined by the fraction unbound (fu) and intrinsic clearance (CL_{int}) (Chapters 4 and 6).

$$CL = fu * CL_{int}$$

Equation 9.2

Combining Equations 1 and 2 and assuming the drug is completely absorbed from the gut ($f_g = 1.0$), the determinants of C_{ss} during chronic dosing are:

$$C_{ss} = \frac{dose\ rate}{fu * CL_{int}}$$

Equation 9.3

Equation 9.3 also applies to high hepatic extraction ratio drugs given orally (Chapter 6).

As F, fu and CL_{int} usually do not change with drug concentration, C_{ss} is directly proportional to dose rate. However, there are some situations where this predictable relationship between dose rate and C_{ss} breaks down due to dose dependency of fu and/or CL_{int}.

Saturation of drug metabolism causing a change in intrinsic clearance

The metabolism of drugs is carried out by a variety of enzymes such as cytochrome P450 and N-acetyltransferase. The dependence of the rate of an enzyme reaction on substrate concentration is given by the Michaelis-Menten equation and is illustrated in Figure 9.1.

$$v = \frac{V_{max} * S}{K_m + S}$$

Equation 9.4

where v is the velocity of reaction, S is the substrate concentration, V_{max} is the maximum velocity at very high substrate concentrations and K_m is the substrate concentration at half V_{max}. K_m is a measure of the affinity of the substrate for the enzyme.

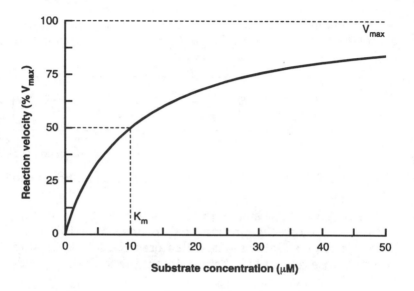

Figure 9.1: Kinetics of drug-metabolising enzymes

Increase in reaction velocity with increase in substrate concentration. As the substrate concentration increases, saturation of substrate binding to the enzyme active site eventually occurs and a maximal reaction velocity (V_{max}) is reached. The substrate concentration at a reaction velocity which is half V_{max} is called the K_m and is a measure of the affinity of the enzyme for the substrate. When substrate concentration is very low compared to K_m, the reaction velocity increases in a linear fashion with substrate concentration. The reaction velocity (v) at any particular substrate concentration (S) is given by:

$$v = \frac{V_{max}*S}{K_m + S}$$

In pharmacokinetic terms, the rate (v) at which the enzyme metabolises the drug is equivalent to the rate of elimination and S is equivalent to the drug concentration (C). From Chapter 1 we saw that:

$$Rate\ of\ elimination = CL*C$$

Equation 9.5

Equation 9.4 can then be rearranged to give a function for intrinsic clearance:

$$CL_{int} = \frac{v}{C} = \frac{V_{max}}{K_m + C}$$

Equation 9.6

where V_{max} is the maximum rate of metabolism at high concentrations of drug and K_m is the drug concentration at half V_{max}.

Usually, plasma drug concentration (C) in the therapeutic range is very small compared to the K_m for the metabolising enzyme and Equation 9.6 approximates to:

$$CL_{int} = \frac{V_{max}}{K_m}$$

Equation 9.7

V_{max} and K_m are constants characteristic of the particular drug substrate and the enzyme metabolising it. CL_{int} is then independent of drug concentration. In some cases, drug concentrations are close to or above K_m at therapeutic doses, and the kinetics begin to become non-linear (see Figure 9.1). In this situation, CL_{int} decreases as drug concentration increases (see Equation 9.6) and steady state drug concentration increases more than proportionately with dose (Equation 9.3). At high drug concentrations, the maximal rate of metabolism is reached and cannot be exceeded. Under these conditions, a constant *amount* of drug is eliminated per unit time no matter how much drug is in the body. Zero order kinetics then apply rather than the usual first order kinetics where a constant *proportion* of the drug in the body is eliminated per unit time. Some examples of drugs which exhibit non-linear kinetic behaviour are phenytoin, ethanol, salicylate and, in some individuals, theophylline.

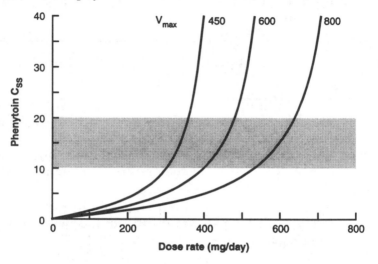

Figure 9.2: Saturation of drug metabolism

Increase in steady state phenytoin concentration with increasing dose rate. In the therapeutic range for phenytoin (10–20 mg/L), small increments in dose cause large increases in plasma phenytoin concentration. The values used for K_m (5 mg/L) and V_{max} (shown) are typical of those found in individuals with epilepsy. The therapeutic range for phenytoin is shown by the shaded area. The function used to generate the data is adapted from Equations 9.3 and 9.6:

$$C_{ss} = \frac{dose\ rate * K_m}{V_{max} - dose\ rate}$$

- *Phenytoin*: Phenytoin exhibits marked saturation of metabolism at concentrations in the therapeutic range (10–20 mg/L) (Figure 9.2). Consequently, small increases in dose result in large increases in total and unbound steady state drug concentration. As an example, for a patient with typical K_m of 5 mg/L (total drug) and V_{max} of 450 mg/day, steady state concentrations at doses of 300, 360 and 400 mg/day would be 10, 20 and 40 mg/L respectively (Figure 9.2). Thus, small dosage adjustments are required to achieve phenytoin concentrations in the therapeutic range of 10–20 mg/L.

A second consequence is that, because clearance decreases, apparent half-life increases from about 12 hours at low phenytoin concentrations to as long as a week or more at high concentrations. This means that:

a) the time to reach steady state can be as long as 1–3 weeks at phenytoin concentrations near the top of the therapeutic range;

b) in the therapeutic range, the phenytoin concentration fluctuates little over a 24-hour period allowing once daily dosing and sampling for drug concentration monitoring at any time between doses;

c) if dosing is stopped with concentrations in the toxic range, phenytoin concentration initially falls very slowly and there may be little change over a number of days.

- *Alcohol*: Alcohol is an interesting example of saturable metabolism. The K_m for alcohol is about 0.01 g% (100 mg/L) so that concentrations in the range of pharmacological effect are well above the K_m. The V_{max} for ethanol metabolism is about 10 g/hour (12.8 mL/hour) and it can be calculated (see legend to Figure 9.2) that at the common legal driving limit of 0.05 g%, the rate of alcohol metabolism per hour is 8.3 g/hour. This amount of alcohol is contained in 530 mL light beer, 236 mL standard beer, 88 mL wine or 27 mL spirit. Higher rates of ingestion will result in further accumulation.

Saturation of first-pass metabolism causing an increase in bioavailability

After oral administration, the drug-metabolising enzymes in the liver are exposed to relatively high drug concentrations in the portal blood during the absorption process. For drugs such as alprenolol with high hepatic extraction ratios, an increased dose can result in saturation of the metabolising enzymes, and a decrease in intrinsic clearance. Steady state drug concentration then increases more than proportionately with dose (Equation 9.3). Other examples of drugs with saturable first-pass metabolism are tropisetron and paroxetine.

Saturation of renal secretion clearance

In Chapter 7, it was shown that renal drug clearance is the sum of filtration clearance plus secretion clearance minus reabsorption. Clearance by glomerular filtration and tubular reabsorption are both passive processes which are not saturable, but secretion involves saturable drug binding to an active transport mechanism. Even when secretion clearance is saturated, filtration clearance continues to increase linearly with plasma drug concentration. The extent to which saturation of renal secretion results in non-linear pharmacokinetics depends on the relative importance of secretion and filtration in the drug's elimination. Because of the baseline of non-saturable filtration clearance, saturation of renal secretion does not usually cause clinically important problems.

Saturation of protein binding sites causing a change in fraction of drug unbound in plasma

From Chapter 8, the fraction unbound of a drug in plasma (fu) is given by

$$fu = \frac{1}{1 + K_a P_u}$$

Equation 9.8

where K_a is the affinity constant for binding to a protein such as albumin or alpha$_1$-acid glycoprotein and P_u is the concentration of free (unbound) protein, that is, protein that does not have drug bound to it. The total concentration of albumin in plasma is about 0.6 mM (40 g/L) and the concentration of alpha$_1$-acid glycoprotein is about 0.015 mM. Usually, drug concentrations are well below those of the binding proteins and unbound protein (P_u) approximates to total protein (P). Then, fu depends only on the affinity constant and the total concentration of protein binding sites, and remains constant with changes in drug concentration. In a few cases (for example, salicylate, phenylbutazone, diflunisal), therapeutic drug concentrations are high enough to saturate albumin binding sites so that unbound protein concentration decreases and fu increases as drug concentration increases. Total drug concentration then increases less than proportionately with increases in dose (Equation 9.3). This occurs more commonly for drugs such as disopyramide which bind to alpha$_1$-acid glycoprotein because of the lower concentration of binding protein.

What are the practical consequences of saturable protein binding? From Equation 9.3, it can be seen that as fu increases, total drug concentration at steady state decreases. However, fu does not affect the steady state concentration of the unbound drug. In other words, unbound concentration will increase proportionately with dose, but total drug concentration will increase less than proportionately. This is illustrated in Figure 9.3 for the case of disopyramide. This dissociation between total and unbound drug concentration causes difficulties in therapeutic drug monitoring where total drug concentration is nearly always measured. Total drug concentration may appear to plateau despite increasing dose (Figure 9.3), leading to the temptation to increase the dose further. However, unbound drug concentrations and drug effect do increase linearly with dose — if this is not realised, inappropriate dose increases with consequent toxicity can occur.

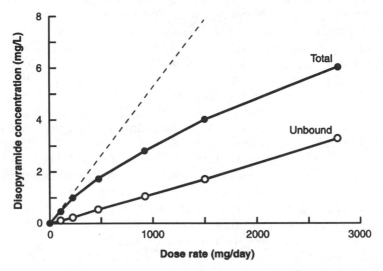

Figure 9.3: Saturation of protein binding

Increase in total and unbound concentrations of disopyramide with dose rate. The increase in unbound concentration is linear with dose, whereas the total concentration increases less than proportionately with dose. The fraction unbound is 0.22 at the lowest concentration and 0.54 at the highest. The dashed line shows how the total concentration would increase with dose if the fraction unbound remained constant at 0.22.

Data used are from P J Meffin et al, *Journal of Pharmacokinetics and Biopharmaceutics* 1979;7:29–46.

? Self-test questions

1. The term linear pharmacokinetics means:
   a) a plot of drug concentration versus time is linear
   b) half-life increases proportionately with dose
   c) a constant amount of drug is eliminated per unit time
   d) clearance is proportional to dose
   e) steady state drug concentration is proportional to dose

2. Which of the following processes are saturable and can result in non-linear pharmacokinetics?
   a) drug metabolism
   b) glomerular filtration
   c) protein binding
   d) renal tubular secretion
   e) renal tubular reabsorption

3. Saturation of drug-metabolising enzymes occurs when:
   a) drug concentration is similar to maximal reaction velocity
   b) the K_m is very high
   c) the drug concentration is above the K_m
   d) the maximal reaction velocity and K_m are similar
   e) the K_m is high compared to the drug concentration

4. Saturation of protein binding occurs when:
   a) the concentration of binding protein is high
   b) the affinity of the drug for the protein is high
   c) the drug concentration approaches the concentration of protein binding sites
   d) fraction unbound (fu) is low
   e) the concentration of protein binding sites is high compared to the drug concentration

5. Regarding alcohol pharmacokinetics:
   a) the K_m for alcohol metabolism is much higher than the concentration causing impairment of driving performance
   b) the maximal velocity of alcohol metabolism in the body is 100 g/hour
   c) at a blood alcohol concentration of 0.05 g% about one standard drink per hour will maintain steady state
   d) in the range of blood alcohol concentrations causing impaired driving performance, alcohol metabolism is saturated
   e) because alcohol metabolism is saturable, blood alcohol concentrations are not a good index of response

10

PHARMACODYNAMICS — THE CONCENTRATION–EFFECT RELATIONSHIP

What is pharmacodynamics?

So far, we have considered how drugs are absorbed, distributed and excreted by the body — the pharmacokinetic phase of drug action. To produce therapeutic or toxic effects, drugs interact with receptors in the body — the pharmacodynamic phase of drug action. The drug in the tissues, where drug–receptor interactions usually occur, is in equilibrium with the unbound drug in the plasma.

How do drugs produce effects?

Drugs usually interact in a structurally specific way with a protein receptor. This activates a second messenger system which produces a biochemical or physiological effect; for example, changes in intracellular calcium concentrations result in muscle contraction or relaxation. The most common receptors are trans-membrane receptors linked to guanosine triphosphate binding proteins (G proteins) which activate second messenger systems such as adenylate cyclase (beta-adrenoreceptors) or the inositol–triphosphate pathway (alpha-adrenoreceptors).

A drug which binds to a receptor and produces a maximum effect is called a full agonist; a drug which binds and produces less than a maximal effect is called a partial agonist. Drugs which bind but do not activate second messenger systems are called antagonists. Antagonists can only produce effects by blocking the access of the natural transmitter (agonist) to the receptor. Thus, beta-blockers produce relatively little change in heart rate when given to subjects at rest as there is low sympathetic tone and little noradrenaline (the natural agonist) to be antagonised at the beta-adrenoreceptor. The effects of betablockers are therefore measured after stimulating the sympathetic nervous system; for example, by measuring the degree to which exercise-induced tachycardia is blocked. Partial agonists produce an effect if no agonist is present, but act as antagonists in the presence of a full agonist. Pindolol, a betablocker which is a partial agonist, produces less decrease in heart rate than pure antagonists such as propranolol.

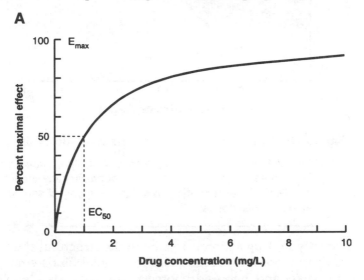

Figure 10.1A: The concentration–effect relationship

A.   The drug concentration–effect relationship is described by the same function as the enzyme velocity–substrate concentration relationship. E is the effect at drug concentration C, E_{max} is the maximal effect at high drug concentrations when all the receptors are occupied by the drug, and EC_{50} is the drug concentration giving half-maximal effect. This is the simplest form of the concentration–effect relationship and more complex expressions are sometimes required to explain the observed effects. The function describing the concentration–effect relationship is:

$$E = \frac{E_{max} * C}{EC_{50} + C}$$

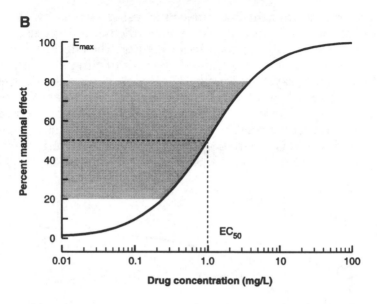

Figure 10.1B: The concentration–effect relationship

B.   When plotted on a semi-logarithmic plot, the curve from Figure 10.1A becomes a sigmoidal shape, but is approximately linear between 20% and 80% of maximal effect, a range commonly observed for drugs used at therapeutic doses.

Selectivity in drug action is related to the structural specificity of drug binding to receptors. Propranolol binds equally well to beta$_1$- and beta$_2$-adrenoreceptors, whereas atenolol and metoprolol bind selectively to and block (are antagonists at) beta$_1$-adrenoreceptors. Salbutamol is a selective beta$_2$-adrenoreceptor agonist and, in this case, additional selectivity is achieved by inhaling the drug directly to its site of action in the lungs.

How does drug effect vary with drug concentration?

The interaction of a drug with a receptor involves it binding to the receptor in the same structurally specific way that a substrate binds to the active site of an enzyme. The same equation and similar parameters are therefore used to describe the concentration–effect relationship (Figure 10.1). Note that this is the same as the expression used in Chapter 9 where it was applied to the interaction of a substrate with a drug-metabolising enzyme. The affinity of the drug for the receptor is described by the EC_{50}, the concentration of the drug required to give half-maximal effect. The different actions of a drug, such as therapeutic and adverse effects, are often due to the drug binding to different receptors with different EC_{50} values. Ideally, adverse effects should occur at higher drug concentrations than therapeutic effects. The ratio adverse effect EC_{50}/ therapeutic effect EC_{50} gives a measure of the safety of the drug and is called the therapeutic index.

Figure 10.1A shows the drug concentration–effect relationship. As drug concentration increases, the effect rises to a maximum, at which point the receptor is saturated. Figure 10.1B shows the curve replotted using a logarithmic concentration (x) axis. Concentration–effect curves are often plotted in this way as the part of the curve between 20% and 80% of maximal effect is approximately linear and this section of the curve most often applies to the action of drugs at therapeutic concentrations. Increasing drug concentration above 80% maximal effect achieves very little in terms of extra therapeutic effects, but increases the risk of adverse effects.

This type of concentration–effect curve is produced by measuring a continuous parameter, such as blood pressure or exercise-induced tachycardia, at various drug concentrations. It is known as a graded concentration–effect curve.

How does effect vary with time after a single dose of a drug?

After a single dose, drug concentration falls in an exponential manner with time — the logarithm of drug concentration is linear with time (see Chapters 2 and 3). From Figure 10.1B, it can be seen that the logarithm of drug concentration is also linear with drug effect in the range 20–80% maximal effect. In this

Pharmacokinetics Made Easy

range, therefore, effect falls in a linear fashion with time (Figure 10.2). If the dose of the drug is large enough to produce a concentration which causes a maximal effect, the effect will change very little until the drug concentration falls to that producing about 80% maximal effect (Figure 10.2). The duration

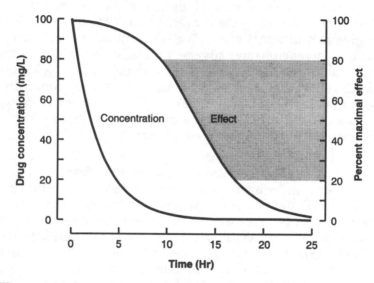

Figure 10.2: The time course of drug concentration and effect after a single dose

Concentration decreases in an exponential manner. If the initial concentration is high enough to be in the region of maximal effect (see Figure 10.1), there is initially little change in effect as the concentration decreases. In this case, as drug concentration falls from 100 mg/L to 4 mg/L, the effect only falls from 99% to 80% of maximal effect. The decrease in effect is then approximately linear with time between 80% and 20% of maximal effect. If the dose had been such that the initial concentration was about 4 mg/L giving about 80% maximal effect, the decrease in effect would have been linear with time from immediately after the dose.

The parameters used were: initial drug concentration (C_0) = 100 mg/L; E_{max} = 100; EC_{50} = 1 mg/L; elimination rate constant k = 0.35/hour (elimination half-life = 2 hours).

of action can be prolonged by increasing the dose, but increases as a logarithmic function of the dose and there is a risk of producing more adverse effects, unless the drug has a large therapeutic index. Beta-blockers are usually given once or twice daily, despite having short elimination half-lives. This is at least partly because they have a large therapeutic index and the doses used are large enough to produce a maximal effect for a significant part of the interval between doses.

How is a therapeutic range (window) defined?

An alternative way of constructing a concentration–effect curve is to determine the percentage of a population of patients showing a defined effect at various drug concentrations. For example, with phenytoin the therapeutic effect might be defined as >80% decrease in the frequency of fits and the adverse effect defined as the proportion of patients developing nystagmus on looking sideways. These are called quantal (population) concentration–effect curves and have the same shape and parameters as the graded concentration–effect curves referred to above.

Figure 10.3 shows quantal (population) concentration–effect curves as they might occur for the therapeutic and adverse effects of phenytoin with a therapeutic concentration range (window) of 10–20 mg/L. At the top of the therapeutic range not all patients will have a therapeutic effect and, within the 'therapeutic range', significant numbers of patients may have adverse effects. As therapeutic ranges are defined on a population basis, they need to be interpreted carefully in relation to individual patients.

When is drug concentration not a good indicator of effect?

- *Drugs used at concentrations which give a maximal effect* (Figure 10.2). For a part of the dose interval, there is no change in effect as concentration decreases. For drugs used at doses giving concentrations in this part of the concentration–effect curve, increasing the dose does not result in an increase in response, but may 'recruit' adverse effects which have separate concentration–effect relationships with higher EC_{50}s (see Figure 10.3).

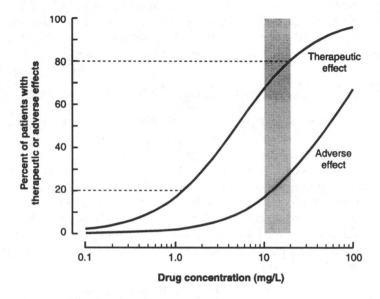

Figure 10.3: Quantal (population) concentration–effect curves and the concept of the therapeutic range (window)

Quantal concentration–effect curves are constructed by determining the cumulative percentage of a patient population with a discrete therapeutic or adverse effect. Such curves are shown for the anticonvulsant phenytoin. Although some patients respond at lower concentrations, the therapeutic range most commonly used is 10–20 mg/L (shaded area), which gives a therapeutic effect (reduction in fit frequency) in most patients with an acceptable incidence of adverse effects (for example, nystagmus, ataxia).

- *'Hit and run' drugs.* Some drugs act irreversibly; for example, the classical monoamine oxidase (MAO) inhibitors or the effect of aspirin on cyclooxygenase in platelets. Termination of these effects relies on synthesis of new MAO or platelets respectively, so that there is no direct relationship between drug concentration and effect.

- *Delayed distribution.* This occurs when the site of drug action is at a site to which the drug is slowly distributed. An example is digoxin (see Chapter 2). The effect *increases* as the drug concentration *falls* due to redistribution. Drug concentrations soon after a dose cause a smaller effect than the same concentrations cause later when distribution to the site of action has occurred. This results in an anticlockwise hysteresis in the concentration–effect relationship (Figure 10.4A).

A

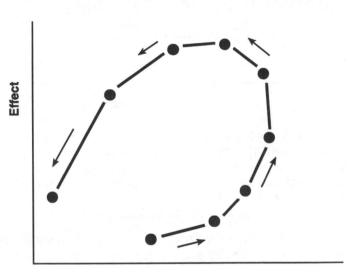

Plasma drug concentration

Figure 10.4: Hysteresis in the concentration–effect relationship

Clockwise and anticlockwise hysteresis loops. The points are concentration–effect measurements made at varying times after a dose. The arrows show the direction of time after the dose.

10.4A. An anticlockwise hysteresis loop occurs when the drug has to be distributed to its site of action. Effect for a given plasma concentration is initially low, but increases as the drug is distributed out of the plasma to the site of action. An example is digoxin.

B

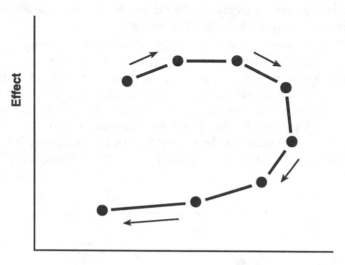

Plasma drug concentration

10.4B. A clockwise hysteresis loop occurs when rapid tolerance (tachyphylaxis) develops. The effect for a given plasma concentration is initially high, but decreases with time after the dose as tolerance rapidly develops. Examples are cocaine or indirectly-acting sympathomimetic drugs such as pseudoephedrine.

- *Acute tolerance (tachyphylaxis).* With some drugs tolerance can occur very rapidly after a single dose. An example of this is the indirectly acting sympathomimetic amines such as amphetamine or ephedrine. These drugs act by releasing noradrenaline from the sympathetic nerve ending which rapidly becomes depleted of neurotransmitter and resistant to further drug effect. Drug concentrations soon after a single dose then cause a greater effect than the same concentrations at a later time. This results in a clockwise hysteresis in the concentration–effect relationship (Figure 10.4B).

- *The 'wrong' effect is measured.* For example, after the first dose the effect of warfarin on prothrombin time increases as the warfarin concentration decreases. The rate of onset of effect is a function of the rate of decay of existing clotting factors. However, the direct effect of warfarin is on the rate of clotting factor synthesis. If this is determined directly, warfarin concentration correlates well with effect.

- *Active metabolites.* If a drug produces active metabolites which contribute to the therapeutic or adverse effects, but are not measured by the analytical method used, there may be an apparent dissociation between concentration and effect. This mechanism can cause an apparent difference between oral and intravenous dosing in the concentration–effect relationship for drugs with high hepatic extraction ratios. After oral dosing, a substantial part of the dose is converted to metabolites during first-pass metabolism so that the dose–effect curve appears shifted to the left compared to intravenous dosing, where plasma concentrations of active metabolites are lower. This effect is seen with several beta-adrenoreceptor antagonists.

- *Enantiomeric drugs.* Many drugs are marketed as racemic mixtures of enantiomers (optical isomers). The enantiomers have essentially identical physico-chemical characteristics, but usually have different pharmacokinetic and pharmacodynamic properties. For example, most beta-adrenoreceptor antagonists are racemic mixtures of two enantiomers with only one of the enantiomers being active. Such drugs are usually measured in plasma by methods which give an answer in terms of the sum of the concentrations of the individual enantiomers. If, as is usually the case, the enantiomers are eliminated at different rates, the ratio between them changes with time resulting in an apparent change in the concentration–effect relationship.

- *Saturable protein binding.* If total (bound plus unbound) drug is measured and the fraction unbound changes with concentration (see Chapter 9), there will be an apparent dissociation between concentration and effect.

? Self-test questions

1. With respect to pharmacodynamics:
   a) a partial agonist can act as either an agonist or an antagonist
   b) a partial agonist requires the presence of a full agonist to produce an effect
   c) the second messenger system for beta-adrenoreceptors is adenylate cyclase
   d) the inositol-triphosphate system is the second messenger for beta-adrenoreceptors
   e) an antagonist requires the presence of an agonist to produce an effect

2. With respect to graded concentration–effect curves:
   a) E_{max} is the drug concentration at maximal effect
   b) EC_{50} is the drug concentration at half maximal effect
   c) when plotted as log concentration versus effect, the curve is approximately linear up to 50% of maximal effect
   d) a drug concentration twice EC_{50} gives an effect that is two-thirds E_{max}
   e) a drug concentration half EC_{50} gives an effect that is one-quarter E_{max}

3. With respect to the time course of drug effect after a single dose:
   a) effect falls in a linear fashion with time over the range 20%–80% of maximal effect
   b) above 80% maximal effect, the drug effect decreases rapidly as drug concentration decreases
   c) doubling the dose doubles the duration of action
   d) doubling the dose normally increases the duration of action by one drug half-life
   e) duration of action is a linear function of dose

4. The therapeutic index:
   a) is the ratio between the maximal therapeutic and toxic effects

b) is the ratio between the EC_{50} for a toxic effect and the EC_{50} for the therapeutic effect

c) depends on the potency of the drug

d) is usually greater than 1

e) refers to the potential to cause allergic drug reactions

5. With respect to drug concentration as an indicator of effect:

a) tachyphylaxis produces a clockwise hysteresis in the concentration–effect relationship

b) delayed distribution to the site of action produces an anti-clockwise hysteresis in the concentration–effect relationship

c) active metabolites cause an apparent shift to the right in the concentration–effect curve

d) drug enantiomers are physico-chemically so similar that they produce the same effects on drug receptors

e) saturable protein binding results in a more than linear increase in unbound drug concentration with dose

11

DESIGNING DOSE REGIMENS

Information from previous chapters can be used to help design dose regimens.

Intravenous infusion and intermittent intravenous bolus dosing

Continuous intravenous infusions and intermittent intravenous boluses are common ways of administering drugs such as gentamicin, lignocaine and theophylline. Figure 11.1 illustrates the plasma concentration time course of theophylline given intravenously. Given as a continuous infusion, the drug accumulates to a steady state concentration (C_{ss}) determined only by the dose rate and clearance (CL) (see Chapter 1). The maintenance dose rate to achieve a target concentration can be calculated if the clearance is known.

$$target\ concentration\ (C_{ss}) = \frac{maintenance\ dose\ rate}{CL}$$

Equation 11.1

The time to reach steady state is determined by the half-life (3–5 half-lives: see Chapter 3).

If intermittent bolus doses are given every half-life (8 hours in this case for theophylline), half the first dose is eliminated over the first dosing interval. Therefore, after the second dose there are 1.5 doses in the body and half of this amount is eliminated before the third dose. The drug continues to accumulate with continued dosing until there is double the dose in the body, at which point the equivalent of one dose is eliminated each dosing interval (half-life). The plasma concentration is then at steady state (rate of administration equals rate of elimination where each is one dose per dosing interval).

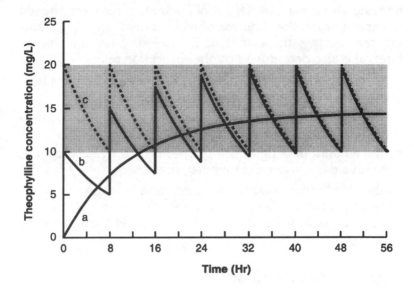

Figure 11.1: Intravenous dosing

Intravenous infusion or intermittent dosing of a drug such as theophylline.

(a) Continuous intravenous infusion at a dose rate of 37.5 mg/hour

(b) Intermittent bolus dosing 300 mg 8-hourly (dose rate (dose/dosing interval) is 37.5 mg/hour)

(c) As for (b) but with a loading dose of 600 mg, twice the maintenance dose

Parameters used in the simulations were: CL = 2.6 L/hour, V = 30 L, $t_{1/2}$ = 8 hours. At steady state, the average plasma concentration over the dosing interval is the same as that during a continuous infusion (14.4 mg/L in this case). The therapeutic range for theophylline is 10–20 mg/L (55–110 mmol/L).

The drug concentration fluctuates over the dosing interval, the maximum concentration being designated C_{max} and the minimum concentration (usually just before the next dose) being designated C_{min}. The extent of the fluctuation with intravenous dosing depends on the ratio of the half-life to the dosing interval — the lower the ratio the greater the fluctuation and vice versa. The degree of fluctuation can be expressed in various ways, the simplest of which is as C_{max}/C_{min}. During oral dosing, the extent of fluctuation over the dosage interval is also determined by the absorption rate (see below).

At steady state during intermittent intravenous bolus dosing with a dosing interval equal to the half-life:

- the plasma concentration fluctuates twofold over the dosing interval;
- the amount of drug in the body shortly after each dose is equivalent to twice the maintenance dose;
- the steady state plasma concentration averaged over the dosing interval ($\overline{C_{ss}}$) is the same as the steady state plasma concentration for a continuous infusion at the same dose rate (see Figure 11.1).

Use of a loading dose

The effect of a loading dose before an intravenous infusion has been discussed in Chapter 2. The loading dose to achieve a target concentration is determined by the volume of distribution (V).

$$loading\ dose = target\ concentration * V$$

Equation 11.2

If the loading dose achieves a plasma drug concentration the same as the steady state concentration for the maintenance infusion (see Equation 11.1), steady state will be immediately achieved and maintained. If the loading dose over- or undershoots the steady state concentration, it will still take 3–5 half-lives to reach C_{ss} (see Chapter 2), but the initial concentration will be closer to the eventual steady state concentration.

With intermittent intravenous bolus dosing, Figure 11.1 shows that where the dosing interval is equal to the half-life of the drug, a loading dose of twice the maintenance dose immediately achieves steady state. Half the loading dose (one maintenance dose) is eliminated in the first dosing interval (one half-life) and is then replaced by the first maintenance dose and so on.

The use of a bolus loading dose may sometimes cause problems if adverse effects occur because of the initial high plasma drug concentrations before redistribution occurs. This is the case, for example, with lignocaine, where central nervous system (CNS) toxicity occurs if too high a loading dose is given too rapidly. In this situation, a loading infusion or series of loading infusions can be used to allow redistribution to occur while the loading dose is being given. A common regimen for lignocaine is to give an initial intravenous dose of 1 mg/kg, followed by up to 3 additional bolus injections of 0.5 mg/kg every 8–10 minutes as necessary, and a maintenance infusion of 2 mg/minute.

Another example is digoxin, where it is common for the loading dose to be divided into 3 parts given at 8-hourly intervals. Digoxin is slowly distributed to its site of action so the full effect of a dose is not seen for about 6 hours (see Chapter 2). Giving the loading dose in parts allows the full effect of each increment to be observed before the next is given so that potential toxicity can be avoided.

Effects of varying the dose interval

So far we have considered a dosing interval equal to the half-life of the drug. Figure 11.2 shows the plasma concentration time profile for once daily intravenous bolus dosing of drugs with half-lives of 6 hours, 24 hours and 96 hours (0.25, 1 and 4 times the dosing interval of 24 hours). For the drug with a half-life of 6 hours (characteristic of theophylline), the concentration is virtually at steady state shortly after the first dose, but there is a large fluctuation (C_{max}/C_{min} = 16) over the dosing interval. The drug with a half-life of 24 hours (characteristic of amitriptyline) takes 3–5 half-lives to reach steady state and the fluctuation over the dosing interval is twofold. For the drug with a half-life of 96 hours (characteristic of phenobarbitone), it takes 12–20 days (3–5 half-lives) to reach steady state, and with once daily dosing (4 doses per half-life), the extent of fluctuation over the dosing interval is small ($C_{max}/C_{min} = 1.2$).

A dosing interval of about a half-life is appropriate for drugs with half-lives of approximately 8–24 hours allowing dosing once, twice or three times daily. It is usually not practicable to administer drugs with shorter half-lives more frequently as compliance with therapy becomes poor with dosing regimens involving complicated and frequent dosing. If a drug with a short half-life has a high therapeutic index, so that a large degree of fluctuation over the dosing interval does not result in toxicity due to high peak concentrations (for example, many antibiotics and beta blocking drugs), it can be given at intervals longer than the half-life. For example, the plasma concentration time profile shown in Figure 11.2A is similar to that for gentamicin when intravenous doses are given 8-hourly (gentamicin half-life is 1–2 hours).

By contrast, if the drug has a low therapeutic index and plasma concentrations need to be maintained in a narrow therapeutic range (for example, theophylline with a therapeutic range of 10–20 mg/L (55–110 mmol/L)), use of a sustained release formulation will be necessary.

If the drug has a very long half-life (for example, phenobarbitone with a half-life of 4 days), once daily administration may still be appropriate and convenient. The fluctuation over the dosing interval will be small, but it should be remembered that it will still take 3–5 half-lives (12–20 days in this example) to reach steady state. A loading dose could be used, but may not be feasible if tolerance to adverse effects occurs as the drug gradually accumulates to steady state. For example, from Equation 11.2, the loading dose of phenobarbitone to reach a plasma concentration of 30 mg/L (in the middle of the therapeutic range for anticonvulsant activity) would be about 1.5 g — a lethal dose for a non-tolerant individual (loading dose = $C*V$ = 30 mg/L x 50 L).

A

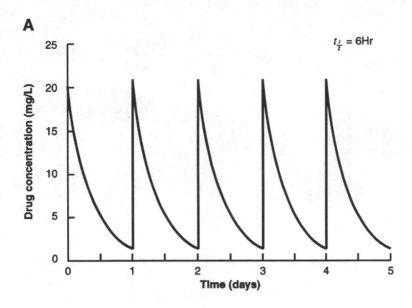

$t_{\frac{1}{2}} = 6Hr$

B

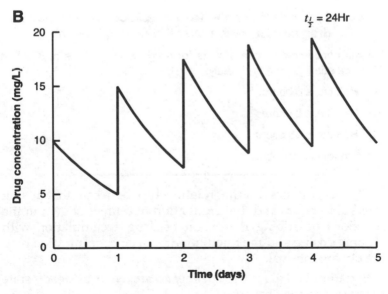

$t_{\frac{1}{2}} = 24Hr$

C

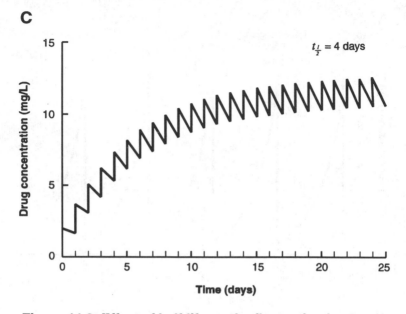

Figure 11.2: Effect of half-life on the fluctuation in plasma drug concentration over the dosing interval

Plasma concentration time profiles for drugs with half-lives of 6, 24 or 96 hours administered once daily:

(A)   Half-life is 6 hours

(B)   Half-life is 24 hours

(C)   Half-life is 96 hours

See text for explanation.

The importance of the relationship between the dosing interval in hours and the elimination half-life is shown in the functions describing the extent of drug accumulation with chronic dosing and the fluctuation in drug concentration over the dosing interval.

Equation 11.3 gives the *extent of accumulation* at steady state compared to the first dose.

$$\frac{C_{max} \text{ steady state}}{C_{max} \text{ first dose}} = \frac{1}{1 - e^{-k\tau}}$$

Equation 11.3

where k is the elimination rate constant (units are per hour; see Chapter 3); and τ is the dosing interval in hours.

Equation 11.4 gives the *extent of fluctuation* over the dosing interval at steady state.

$$\frac{C_{max} \text{ steady state}}{C_{min} \text{steady state}} = \frac{1}{e^{-k\tau}}$$

Equation 11.4

In both cases it is the relationship between dosing interval and elimination half-life that is the determinant as

$$-k\tau = -\frac{0.693\tau}{t_{\frac{1}{2}}}$$

Equation 11.5

Oral dosing

The principles applying to intermittent intravenous dosing also apply to oral dosing with two differences (Figure 11.3):

- The slower absorption of oral doses 'smoothes' the plasma concentration profile so that fluctuation over the dosing interval is less than with intravenous bolus dosing. This smoothing effect is exaggerated with sustained release formulations (see Chapter 3 and Figure 3.3), allowing less frequent administration for drugs with short half-lives.

- The dose reaching the systemic circulation is affected by the bioavailability so that at steady state

$$target\ concentration\ (C_{ss}) = \frac{F * oral\ dose\ rate}{CL}$$

Equation 11.6

where F is the bioavailability (compare with Equation 11.1 and see Chapter 5). The relationship between oral and intravenous dose rates to achieve the same C_{ss} is then (combining Equations 11.1 and 11.6)

$$oral\ dose\ rate = \frac{intravenous\ dose\ rate}{F}$$

Equation 11.7

For example, the oral bioavailability of theophylline is close to complete ($F = 1$), so that oral and intravenous dose rates are about the same. Morphine has an oral bioavailability of about 0.2 due to extensive first-pass metabolism, so to achieve similar plasma concentrations and clinical effects, oral dose rates need to be about 5 times intravenous dose rates (intravenous dose rate/0.2).

Other routes of administration and special dose forms also need to be considered. Parenteral dosing by the intramuscular or subcutaneous routes will give absorption profiles similar to those seen with oral dosing. Absorption from intramuscular sites can be very slow for some drugs, such as phenytoin and diazepam, and can be erratic if tissue blood flow is disturbed as in shock. Sustained release parenteral formulations (depot formulations) of antipsychotic drugs, for example, are used to give slow (but sometimes variable) absorption over weeks to months from an intramuscular depot injection allowing infrequent dosing and ensuring compliance.

Transdermal administration of drugs such as glyceryl trinitrate, nicotine or oestrogens avoids first-pass metabolism and provides a slow absorption rate imposed by the rate of transfer through the skin or the release rate of the patch formulation.

Summary

The intravenous loading dose is determined by the volume of distribution:

$$loading\ dose = target\ concentration * V$$

Equation 11.8

The oral maintenance dose rate is determined by the clearance, bioavailability and the target steady state plasma concentration:

$$maintenance\ dose\ rate\ =\ \frac{CL * C_{ss}}{F}$$

Equation 11.9

The time to reach steady state is determined by the elimination half-life:

$$time\ to\ steady\ state = 3\text{--}5\ half\text{-}lives$$

Equation 11.10

The degree of plasma concentration fluctuation over the dosing interval is determined by:
- the half-life
- the absorption rate
- the dosing interval

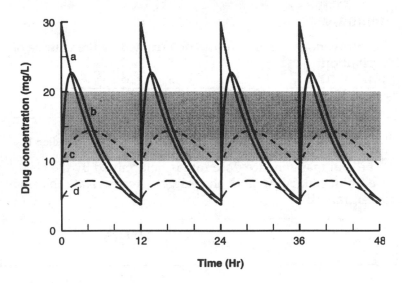

Figure 11.3: Effects of absorption rate and bioavailability on the plasma drug concentration–time profile over the dose interval

The example is characteristic of theophylline in children, who metabolise the drug more quickly than adults. Note the effect of the sustained release preparation in reducing the degree of fluctuation over the dosing interval and allowing 12-hourly dosing for a drug with a short half-life and narrow therapeutic index (therapeutic range 10–20 mg/L (55–110 mmol/L)). The k_a is the absorption rate constant (a measure of the rate of absorption in the same way that the elimination rate constant is a measure of rate of elimination).

Parameters used in the simulations were:

Dose rate = 13 mg/kg/12 hours (1.08 mg/kg/hour), V = 0.5 L/kg, $t_{1/2}$ = 4 hours, CL = 0.086 L/hour/kg, F = 1

(a)   instantaneous absorption (intravenous bolus dosing)

(b) k_a = 1.5 per hour similar to a rapidly absorbed oral formulation

(c) k_a = 0.15 per hour similar to a sustained release formulation

(d)   as for (c) except that bioavailability (F) = 0.5

From Equation 11.6:

for (a), (b) and (c), C_{ss} is 12.6 mg/L and

for (d), C_{ss} is 6.3 mg/L due to reduced bioavailability.

? Self-test questions

1. During a constant rate intravenous infusion, the steady state drug concentration is determined by:
   a) the half-life
   b) the clearance
   c) the dose rate
   d) the volume of distribution
   e) the loading dose

2. A loading dose at the start of a constant rate intravenous infusion:
   a) increases the steady state drug concentration
   b) gets to steady state more quickly
   c) starts closer to the steady state drug concentration
   d) allows a lower infusion rate
   e) always achieves steady state immediately

3. With respect to intermittent intravenous dosing with a dosing interval equal to the half-life of the drug:
   a) it takes one half-life to reach steady state
   b) a loading dose equal to the maintenance dose achieves steady state immediately
   c) it takes 3–5 half-lives to reach steady state
   d) a loading dose of twice the maintenance dose achieves steady state immediately
   e) at steady state an amount of drug equal to the maintenance dose is eliminated during each dosing interval

4. During intermittent intravenous dosing the fluctuation in plasma drug concentration over the dosing interval:
   a) for a given drug half-life, becomes larger as the dosing interval increases
   b) for a given drug half-life, becomes smaller as the frequency of dosing decreases
   c) is twofold if the dosing interval equals the drug half-life
   d) for a given dosing interval, increases as the drug half-life increases

  e) depends on the ratio of the drug half-life to the dosing interval

5. During oral dosing, C_{max}/C_{min} is determined by:
  a) the elimination half-life
  b) the loading dose
  c) the absorption rate
  d) the dosing interval
  e) the average drug concentration over the dosing interval

12

THERAPEUTIC DRUG MONITORING

What is therapeutic drug monitoring?

Therapeutic drug monitoring refers to the individualisation of dosage by maintaining plasma or blood drug concentrations within a target range (therapeutic range, therapeutic window). There are two major sources of variability between individual patients in drug response. These are variation in the relationship between:

- dose and plasma concentration (pharmacokinetic variability)
- drug concentration at the receptor and the drug effect (pharmacodynamic variability).

This is illustrated in Figure 12.1.

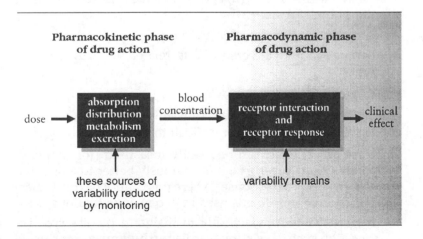

Figure 12.1: Pharmacokinetics and pharmacodynamics

By adjusting doses to maintain plasma drug concentrations within a target range, variability in the pharmacokinetic phase of drug action is greatly reduced. The major sources of pharmacokinetic variability are shown in Table 12.1.

Table 12.1: Major sources of pharmacokinetic variability

Compliance
Age — neonates, children, elderly
Physiology — gender, pregnancy
Disease — hepatic, renal, cardiovascular, respiratory
Drug interactions
Environmental influences on drug metabolism
Genetic polymorphisms of drug metabolism

For which drugs is monitoring helpful?

The characteristics of drugs which make therapeutic drug monitoring useful are:

- marked pharmacokinetic variability
- therapeutic and adverse effects related to drug concentration
- narrow therapeutic index
- defined therapeutic (target) concentration range
- desired therapeutic effect difficult to monitor.

If the clinical effect can be readily measured (for example, heart rate, blood pressure), it is obviously better to adjust the dose on the basis of response. Where this cannot be done, therapeutic drug monitoring is used in two major situations:

- drugs used prophylactically to maintain the *absence* of a condition such as seizures, cardiac arrhythmias, depressive or manic episodes, asthma relapses or organ rejection

- to avoid serious toxicity as with the aminoglycoside antibiotics which, unlike most antibiotics, have a narrow therapeutic range.

Table 12.2: Drugs commonly monitored

Drug	Therapeutic range (mg/L)
Digoxin	0.5–2.0 (microgram/L)
Amiodarone	1.0–2.5
Lignocaine	2.0–5.0
Quinidine	2.0–5.0
Flecainide	0.2–0.9
Mexilitine	0.5–2.5
Salicylate	150–300
Perhexiline	0.15–0.6
Theophylline	10–20
Phenytoin	10–20
Carbamazepine	5–12
Sodium valproate	50–100
Phenobarbitone	15–40
Gentamicin, tobramycin, netilmicin	trough <2[1]; peak > 5
Amikacin	trough <5[1]; peak >15
Vancomycin	trough <10; peak 20–40
Lithium	0.5–1.0 (mmol/L)

1. Recommendations for 8-hourly dosing. Aminoglycosides are increasingly dosed once daily in most but not all situations. Once daily dosing maintains therapeutic effect, probably due to a post-antibiotic effect, but toxicity is reduced. Trough levels of 2 mg/L are too high for once daily dosing, but firm guidelines for therapeutic monitoring are not currently available. The major determinant of toxicity is duration of therapy due to slow accumulation of aminoglycosides in the perilymph and endolymph of the inner ear and in the proximal tubule cells of the renal tubule.

A list of drugs for which therapeutic drug monitoring is commonly used is shown in Table 12.2 with the target or therapeutic ranges. The ranges used are in most cases derived from observation of therapeutic and adverse effects in small groups of patients. Therefore, when applied to a wider population of patients, there will be individuals who achieve adequate effects at lower concentrations or experience adverse events within the 'therapeutic range'. There are two major important principles in using therapeutic ranges:

- Most drug responses are graded responses and are continuous through the concentration range (see Chapter 10). Therapeutic responses do not magically 'switch on' at the lower limit of the therapeutic range, nor do toxic responses suddenly appear at the upper limit.
- Individual patients will have individual therapeutic ranges — this is the residual pharmacodynamic variability in Figure 12.1.

Sampling and drug analysis

Assay methods

Drug assay methods should have adequate sensitivity, be specific for the drug (or metabolite) to be measured and have appropriate accuracy and precision. Most high-volume drug assays are now carried out by automated immunoassay methods which have these characteristics. However, a number continue to require manual assay by methods such as high performance liquid chromatography (HPLC) and gas liquid chromatography (GLC) (for example, amiodarone, perhexiline). National and international quality control programs are available for most commonly monitored drugs, and reputable laboratories are accredited by organisations such as the National Association of Testing Authorities.

Sample collection

Usually, plasma or serum is used for drug assays, depending on the equipment used. However, with cyclosporin there are large shifts of drug between red cells and plasma with storage and temperature change, so whole blood is assayed. Some blood collecting tubes, especially those containing a gel to separate cells and plasma, may not be suitable for all drugs due to drug adsorption by the gel or other components in the tube.

Timing of samples

The correct time of sampling is important. Drug concentrations vary over the dosing interval and with the duration of dosing in relation to achieving a steady state (see Chapter 11). This is unlike most physiological parameters, such as serum creatinine or serum sodium, which change relatively slowly.

The least variable point in the dosing interval is the pre-dose or trough concentration. For drugs with short half-lives in relation to the dosing interval, samples should be collected pre-dose. For drugs with long half-lives, such as phenytoin, phenobarbitone or amiodarone, samples collected at any point in the dosage interval can be satisfactory. For digoxin, any point after the distribution phase (after 6 hours post-dose — see Chapter 2) is acceptable. It should also be remembered that therapeutic ranges have often been established using trough concentrations. Allowance will have to be made if samples are taken at other points in the dosage interval.

As outlined in Chapters 2, 3 and 11, the approach to steady state is determined by the half-life and the use, or not, of a loading dose. It is usually best to wait until steady state has been reached before taking a blood sample for assay unless there are concerns about toxicity. This does not apply to drugs such as amiodarone and perhexiline with very long half-lives and which can cause severe toxicity — steady state may take months to be reached and dose adjustments need to be made along the way. With all drugs, if a sample is taken before steady state is reached, allowance needs to be made for this in interpreting the drug concentration.

What information is required for interpretation?

Drug concentrations need to be interpreted in the context of the individual patient without rigid adherence to a therapeutic range.

The basic information about the sample and the patient required for adequate interpretation of a drug concentration is shown in Table 12.3. Besides this, a good knowledge of the disposition of the drug is needed.

Table 12.3: Information required for interpretation of plasma drug concentrations

Time of sample in relation to last dose
Duration of treatment with the current dose
Dosing schedule
Age, gender of patient
Other drug therapy
Relevant disease states particularly renal and hepatic
Reason for request — for example, lack of effect, routine monitoring, suspected toxicity

There are two important factors which can make interpretation of a result difficult in some cases. These are changes in protein binding and active metabolites.

Protein binding

Assays are done using plasma or blood and thus measure total (bound and unbound) drug, whereas it is the unbound drug that interacts with the receptor to produce a response. If binding is changed by disease states, displacement by another drug or non-linearity in protein binding, the interpretation of total plasma or blood drug concentrations must be modified (Chapter 8).

For example, the therapeutic range for phenytoin based on total drug concentration is 10–20 mg/L which corresponds to an unbound drug concentration of 1–2 mg/L (fraction unbound, fu, is normally 0.1). If fu is increased to 0.2, as, for example, in renal disease, the target unbound concentration is still 1–2 mg/L, but the therapeutic range for total drug is 5–10 mg/L. Unless this is realised, inappropriate dose adjustments may be made, resulting in toxicity.

Sodium valproate and salicylate show non-linear binding in the therapeutic range, making interpretation of total drug concentrations difficult (see Chapter 9).

Active metabolites

Metabolites which may not be measured can contribute to the therapeutic response. Examples include carbamazepine (carbamazepine-10,11-epoxide), and procainamide (N-acetyl-procainamide). Theophylline in neonates (but not in adults) is converted to caffeine, so the therapeutic range for theophylline in neonatal apnoea is 6–12 mg/L (allowing for the contribution of caffeine), whereas it is 10–20 mg/L for obstructive airways disease in adults. The therapeutic ranges for imipramine and amitriptyline are based on the combined concentrations of parent drug and active metabolite (desipramine and nortriptyline respectively). Finally, primidone treatment is monitored by measuring the concentration of the active metabolite phenobarbitone, but primidone itself and another metabolite, phenylethylmalonamide, are also active.

Dose forecasting

Several methods have been developed to improve the prediction of individual dose requirements based on sparse data for individual patients. These are based either on calculation of clearance and volume of distribution from one or a few timed drug concentrations, or by a Bayesian feedback method. This latter method is based on differences between 'typical' population parameter values and those predicted for the individual patient from measured drug concentrations.

Is monitoring cost-effective?

Therapeutic drug monitoring is now so taken for granted that the difficulties in managing some drugs without it are forgotten. While the digoxin therapeutic range is somewhat 'loose', the advent of monitoring resulted in a far greater appreciation of the toxicity of digoxin and the need for rational dosing. Similarly, theophylline, while now falling out of favour for other reasons, was rescued from oblivion when the advent of therapeutic drug monitoring in the 1970s allowed its use largely without the serious toxicity previously associated with it. The use of any of the drugs in Table 12.2 without monitoring would be difficult and often dangerous. Emphasis should be placed not so much on whether monitoring is necessary as on how to use it in the most cost-effective and clinically effective manner possible.

? Self-test questions

1. The therapeutic range:
   a) is determined by the clearance of the drug
   b) removes pharmacodynamic variability
   c) must be adhered to in all patients
   d) removes pharmacokinetic variability
   e) varies between patients

2. Regarding the therapeutic drug monitoring of phenytoin:
   a) the therapeutic range is 10–20 mg/L
   b) samples can be taken at any time in the dose interval
   c) free (unbound) phenytoin must always be measured
   d) phenytoin pharmacokinetics are non-linear in the therapeutic range
   e) the therapeutic range based on free (unbound) phenytoin concentrations should be altered for renal failure patients

3. Which of the following drugs have active metabolites which can contribute to their therapeutic effect?
   a) phenytoin

b) carbamazepine
c) primidone
d) gentamicin
e) amitriptyline

4. Regarding the therapeutic drug monitoring of digoxin:
   a) samples should be taken within 6 hours of a dose
   b) steady state is reached within 2 days
   c) the therapeutic concentration range is 0.5–2 mg/L
   d) concentrations above 2 microgram/L invariably indicate toxicity
   e) samples taken at times greater than 6 hours after a dose are satisfactory

5. Regarding samples for therapeutic drug monitoring:
   a) pre-dose (trough) samples are generally the most satisfactory
   b) samples for digoxin should be taken exactly 6 hours post-dose
   c) for cyclosporin measurement whole blood is better than plasma
   d) samples for steady state phenobarbitone monitoring can be taken 4 days after starting treatment
   e) a lithium–heparin tube should be used when taking samples for lithium therapeutic drug monitoring

ANSWERS

Chapter 1
1. b, d
2. c, d
3. b, c, d
4. a, c

Chapter 2
1. d
2. c, d
3. b, d
4. a

Chapter 3
1. a, c, d
2. c, d, e
3. d
4. e
5. b, d, e

Chapter 4
1. a, d
2. b
3. b, d
4. b, c, e
5. b

Chapter 5
1. c, d
2. c
3. a, c
4. b
5. a, b, e

Chapter 6
1. b, d
2. a
3. a, d
4. d
5. c

Chapter 7
1. b
2. b, d, e
3. b, c, d
4. b, d, e
5. b, d, e

Chapter 8
1. a, c
2. a, c, e
3. b, e
4. a, b
5. c, e

Chapter 9
1. e
2. a, c, d
3. c
4. c
5. c, d

Chapter 10
1. a, c, e
2. b, d
3. a, d
4. b, d
5. a, b

Chapter 11
1. b, c
2. c
3. c, d, e
4. a, c, e
5. a, c, d

Chapter 12
1. d, e
2. a, b, d
3. b, c, e
4. e
5. a, c